Wall Pilates For Seniors

Toni Avalos

Table of Contents

Find Resources and Support at:

StrongandAgeless.com

SCAN ME

Introduction

Approaching your senior years can often be fraught with challenges. The last thing you want is to find yourself wading through all the latest fitness fads, trying to decide which ones are best suited to your maturing physique!

You may have heard about Wall Pilates from a friend, social media, or possibly on the news. At first, you were probably skeptical. After all, how do you know that Wall Pilates is as simple as it looks in the adverts and clips? And even more importantly, are other seniors even attempting it or succeeding at it? This is the precise reason this guide on Wall Pilates was published and aimed at seniors who want to get their foot in the door (or on the wall, I should say!)

The most important snippet of information you need before we leap into the *what-and-how* of this incredible exercise format is that it is perfectly suited to senior physiques of all shapes and sizes.

Most of its success with people in our age group is the stability the wall provides during each exercise, ensuring that each movement is controlled, poised, and precisely working the right muscle every time. That means less wasted time flailing and wobbling around while trying to get movements right. And it also means better results from the very first week.

Of course, there's even more to it than that. While Wall Pilates ensures guided movements with proper body alignment and posture while maximizing effectiveness, it also minimizes the risk of injury. That's because Wall Pilates uses your own body weight and strength, along with the support and rigidity of the wall, to ensure that each exercise you do is precise, safe, and within your handling capacity.

Wall Pilates is one of the most effective low-impact exercises to trim down, tone up, and build strong, lean muscle. Add to that, it has a reputation for reducing neck, back, and joint pain. All you need to get started is... a wall! If you want to be comfortable, add an exercise mat, stretchy clothing, and a water bottle.

If you're ready to enjoy improved flexibility, improved range of motion, mobility and independence while exercising safely, you've picked up just the right book. In the pages to follow, you'll enjoy easy-to-follow instructions paired with simple illustrations to help you get started.

This book takes the guesswork out of it.

Chapter 1:

What is Wall Pilates?

What is Wall Pilates?

You're bound to be wondering what Wall Pilates is all about. Where does it originate from? And how does it compare to regular Pilates? Pilates is not a new concept. You've probably already encountered it or have some understanding of it. Pilates is a low-impact exercise focusing on strengthening muscles while improving flexibility and posture. Core muscles are the focal point in this type of exercise, but you can expect to work out your lower legs, glutes, and arms, too. Basic equipment used in Pilates includes a mat, different-sized balls, handled rings, blocks, ankle weights, and more.

How Does it Compare to Pilates?

Wall Pilates is a variation of regular Pilates that uses wall resistance and body weight to strengthen muscles and boost flexibility. You won't need any equipment to do Wall Pilates except for a wall and an exercise mat. The wall supports stretching and toning, which also provides stability to ensure each slow and controlled movement is correctly carried out.

Who Came Up With Pilates?

Who is the brains behind Pilates? First prize for creating Pilates and promoting it somewhat effectively is none other than Joseph Hubertus Pilates, who lived sometime between 1883 and 1967. Yes, Pilates is that old! He didn't just get people on board with Pilates but came up with the concept himself, which isn't surprising, considering he was a German inventor, writer, and physical trainer seemingly obsessed with physical fitness!

Rumor has it that Pilates was born in Dusseldorf and was, for the most part, a sickly child. He became obsessed with becoming stronger and fitter, and so started bodybuilding as a teen. He was quite good at it because he was getting modeling contract offers by the time he hit his teens! Some say that he spent all his time researching and trying out all forms of exercise, eventually settling on a mix of Eastern and Western fitness.

To understand just how sporty Pilates was, you'd need to learn that by the age of 32, he was already a pro boxer, diver, and skier. He even went on to teach self-defense to detectives in Scotland Yard and become an acrobat for the circus. Long story short, if you're following the teachings of Pilates, you're in good hands! Its creator was all that and a whole lot more when it came to health and fitness.

Pilates created Pilates during the First World War when the British interned him as a German enemy alien. His idea was to develop a body conditioning exercise format, and we all know he succeeded!

Just How Effective is Pilates?

Pilates has several scientifically proven benefits. For starters, Pilates promotes strength and mobility in all major muscle groups. It does this with a balanced approach while focusing on deep core muscles. While doing that, it also improves balance, strength, flexibility, posture, and body awareness. Just how effective is Pilates? Very! To illustrate the point, here's a brief look at the benefits of Pilates:

Boosts Core Strength

Most of us don't give our core a second thought... until we find a reason to use it and then realize just how weak it is! Sedentary lifestyles can be common for seniors; that does nothing for core strength. A weak core leads to health issues, such as back pain, instability, and the inability to lift and carry heavy things. The core consists of more than just the stomach muscles – it also includes the back and sides.

Wall Pilates is a great way to boost the strength of deep abdominal muscles while improving posture. While doing Wall Pilates, the wall provides added stability for the spine, keeping everything firmly in place while you focus on correct movements that engage the deep abdominal muscles. Without the wall, you may find yourself wobbling around, getting tired quickly, or even doing the movements wrong, which puts you at risk of injury.

Kickstarts Muscle Strength and Endurance

Exercise is only effective if the workout is having an impact on your muscles. Developing muscle endurance is important because it means that your muscles can carry out repetitive movements for a long time. In short, staying power! Muscle strength and endurance are about more than just being able to do 20-odd reps of each exercise at the gym. It comes into play in everyday life, like carrying groceries from the car to the house or lifting your grandchildren to hug them. Wall Pilates boosts muscle strength and endurance through controlled, slow, and definitive movements. As your strength builds, you can increase the time under tension, thus building and developing more strength and endurance. It's a cycle – a good one!

Boosts Flexibility

Flexibility and fitness don't always go hand in hand. Those are things that comes with consistency. Technically speaking, developing flexibility involves training the muscles regularly to stretch, which causes them to become less taught and loosen up. At the same time, the muscle starts to elongate. This is why you may not be able to touch your toes today, but if you practice stretching correctly for a week, you may get closer to your toes. The trick to maintaining flexibility is consistency!

Wall Pilates requires a series of slow, steady movements, most of which involve stretching of some kind. This improves flexibility while building muscle. Using the wall, you can deepen stretches and increase your range of motion while ensuring you carry out each movement and stretch correctly.

Easy on Joints

One of the biggest gripes of seniors is aches and pains. Joint pain can be a real buzzkill, especially if it's at a point where it's impacting your everyday life. Exercise is a great way to ease joint pain, but many forms of exercise are high impact and exert force on the joints, worsening the problem. Exercises like Pilates are low-impact and designed to strengthen the muscles surrounding joints, thus providing them with more blood flow and joints. There's certainly a reason why Pilates is considered an excellent form of rehab exercise after injury.

Pilates improves core strength while enhancing muscular endurance and flexibility – all great for taking the load off your joints. The wall in Wall Pilates is used as a stabilizer, ensuring you can ease yourself into challenging positions that would otherwise seem impossible. Now that you've got a bit more insight into the basics of Wall Pilates and its benefits let's dig a little deeper into the reasons why Wall Pilates is so well suited to seniors.

Chapter 2:

Pillars of Power

Building the Foundation

Choosing an exercise to commit your time and attention comes down to what it's all about and whether it's a good choice for you. That's why I love telling people that at the heart of Wall Pilates lies a set of principles that form the foundation for its practice, and they're often referred to as the "Pillars of Power." For people like me, these pillars of power are impressive. Wall Pilates for seniors uses the same fundamental principles as Pilates but with a twist (don't worry – the twist isn't a painful one!) These principles include:

Breathing Correctly

The principle of breathing is a vital pillar in the realm of Wall Pilates. Joseph Pilates emphasized that breathing is the most crucial part of exercise and recognized the intrinsic connection between breath and movement. Wall Pilates features rhythmic, deliberate breathing techniques. This doesn't refer to the puffing and panting of exertion, but rather the deep dedicated breathing that facilitates physical exertion instead of exacerbating it. And this contributes to a deeper mind-body connection.

The breathing format in Wall Pilates is not merely a physiological necessity but a tool for enhancing the effectiveness of each exercise. Deep diaphragmatic breathing is encouraged, promoting the engagement of the core muscles and fostering a sense of control. As you synchronize your breath with movements, you create a seamless flow that enhances the fluidity of exercises. This synchronized breath not only oxygenates the body but also allows you to activate key muscle groups, particularly those in the core.

The breath serves as a guide for movement, setting the pace for each exercise. Inhales often precede preparatory movements, while exhales coincide with the exertion phase of an exercise. This intentional coordination allows you to move with precision and control, maximizing the benefits of each movement. The emphasis on breath aligns with the broader goal of Wall Pilates, which is to create a mindful and intentional approach to exercise.

The rhythmic ebb and flow of breath in Wall Pilates contribute to a meditative quality within the practice. Note, I said *meditative quality*. It's not essentially the act of meditation – unless you want it to be, of course. As you focus on the inhalation and exhalation, you enter a state of mindfulness and deeper concentration. Think of it as an inner vehicle that allows you to achieve an inner focus and rhythm. This meditative quality distinguishes Wall Pilates from more strenuous forms of physical activity, transforming it into a holistic practice that nurtures both the body and the mind.

Proper breathing in Wall Pilates extends beyond the workout, promoting a heightened awareness of breath in everyday life. The controlled, rhythmic breath cultivated in Wall Pilates can be applied to manage stress, release tension, enhance focus, and promote relaxation. This integration of breath awareness into daily life reflects the transformative power of Wall Pilates, extending its benefits beyond the confines of a workout session.

Control

If you feel you're not entirely in control of the aging process, you're not. But that doesn't mean that you can't get any sense of control in some shape and form. And that's where Wall Pilates comes in. With Wall Pilates, you can have some control over how your body handles the aging process in terms of strength, endurance, and available energy.

Control is a core pillar of Wall Pilates, and it involves performing each exercise deliberately, controlled, and consciously. Joseph Pilates believed in mind over matter, where your body obeys your will, not your mood or the mood of someone else. This principle's heart is the meticulous regulation of movement, demanding precision and coordination in every exercise. Control is a means to cultivate a profound connection between the mind and body, elevating Pilates beyond a physical workout to a holistic practice encompassing mental discipline and concentration.

The engagement of the core muscles is central to the concept of control in Wall Pilates. The deep abdominals, pelvic floor, and back muscles are pivotal in maintaining stability and executing precise movements. You build physical strength and enhance overall body awareness by consciously activating these muscles. Such engagement also serves as a protective mechanism, promoting proper alignment and reducing the risk of injury.

Wall Pilates distinguishes itself from other forms of exercise by emphasizing control. It's not about the quantity of repetitions but the quality of each movement. Your goal should be to move deliberately focus on maintaining precisely control throughout each exercise, from start to finish. This deliberate approach fosters a mindful connection between the body and mind, creating awareness that extends beyond the Wall Pilates exercise into daily life.

Control in Wall Pilates also extends from physical to mental discipline. As you navigate through the various exercises, you must concentrate on the intricacies of each movement. The concentration required during Wall Pilates sessions contributes to improved cognitive function, stress reduction, and a heightened sense of well-being.

In Wall Pilates, control isn't rigid but is somewhat fluid and adaptable. Wall Pilates encourages you to move with control through a full range of motion, and this essentially promotes flexibility and suppleness. It challenges you to be in command of your body in different positions and situations, fostering a sense of confidence and competence. As you refine your control in Wall Pilates, you build a strong and resilient body and embark on a journey towards greater self-awareness and mastery of body and mind.

Centering Yourself

If you've ever felt a bit wobbly on your feet or off balance as you age, you'll know just how important it is to feel centred. This keeps us balanced and feeling as if we're headed in the right direction, with stability, that is!

Centering happens to be another pillar of Pilates, emphasizing the importance of locating and maintaining a robust and stable center, often called the "powerhouse." You can't generate power from a position of instability, and increasing core stability is one of the benefits of most Pilate programs.

The powerhouse in Wall Pilates comprises the muscles of the lower back, abdomen, buttocks, and hips. It is the focal point from which all movements originate and radiate. By anchoring movements from the center, you can establish a solid foundation for every exercise, promoting stability, balance, and control.

Centering is not solely about physical strength. It also involves an intricate awareness of the body's alignment and engagement. Through a series of stretching movements designed to activate and strengthen the muscles of the powerhouse, you can develop a heightened sense of core stability. This stability, in turn, contributes to improved posture and spinal alignment.

The centering concept goes beyond the physical domain, extending to mental focus and concentration. As you engage your powerhouse, you're encouraged to maintain a deep sense of concentration, ensuring that each movement is executed with precision and control.

Without the wall to lean on, you'd undoubtedly be doing a bit of wincing and flailing around. But with focus and the wall to provide added stability, centering is possible, which brings a whole new dynamic to the exercise.

This mental aspect of centering reinforces the mind-body connection, turning Wall Pilates into a mindful practice that fosters a holistic approach to health and fitness.

Centering is particularly transformative for individuals seeking to address issues related to spinal health. By improving the strength of muscles surrounding the spine and promoting proper alignment, Wall Pilates through centering becomes an effective tool for preventing and alleviating back pain. The emphasis on core strength and stability extends to the entire body, creating a ripple effect that enhances overall strength and flexibility.

Moreover, centering in Wall Pilates is dynamic since it requires constant engagement and mindfulness throughout each exercise. Whether performing a simple abdominal curl or a more complex movement, the awareness of the powerhouse remains constant. This dynamic engagement builds physical resilience and cultivates a sense of self-awareness that carries over into daily life.

Precision

Precision embodies deliberate movement, emphasizing accuracy and meticulous attention to detail. Joseph Pilates envisioned his method as a system that prioritizes quality over quantity, and precision is the key to unlocking the full potential of each exercise.

In Wall Pilates, precision is reflected in the careful alignment of the body and the intentional activation of specific muscle groups. Each movement is designed with a purpose, and you're encouraged to execute exercises with exactitude. Precision is not about rushing through the motions but about performing each exercise deliberately, ensuring that the body is in the optimal position for maximum benefit.

Emphasizing precision transforms Wall Pilates into a mindful and meditative experience that requires you to be fully present in the moment. Precision is particularly crucial in preventing injury and promoting balanced muscle development. You can target specific muscle groups by executing movements precisely and avoid unnecessary strain on joints and ligaments. This careful approach to movement is especially beneficial for older individuals, people recovering from injuries or those seeking a low-impact yet effective exercise method.

Precision in Wall Pilates serves to refine movement patterns, creating a sense of grace and fluidity. Each exercise is a choreographed sequence that demands attention to form and control. Through deliberate movement, you can build physical strength while cultivating a sense of poise and elegance in your approach to exercise.

As you progress through the Wall Pilates journey, precision becomes a guiding principle in every aspect of your life. Your attention to detail extends to daily activities, promoting mindful movement and conscious posture. Precision in Wall Pilates thus becomes a transformative force, shaping the body and instilling a sense of alertness and attention to detail that carries over into various facets of life.

Concentration

The concentration pillar in Wall Pilates serves as the gateway to movement mastery. Joseph Pilates recognized the intricate connection between the mind and body, and concentration is a critical principle that elevates Wall Pilates beyond physical exercise to a holistic practice that nurtures mental focus and awareness.

In Wall Pilates, concentration refers to the focused attention and intentional mental engagement required during each exercise. While performing each exercise, you're encouraged to be fully present in the moment, immersing yourself in the intricacies of each movement, where the mind and body collaborate in a dance of awareness.

The mindful movement cultivated through concentration is about executing precise physical movements and understanding the nuances of how the body responds to each exercise. Concentrating on the sensations, breath, and alignment can deepen your connection with your body, fostering a heightened body awareness that extends to daily life.

Concentration in Wall Pilates is closely interwoven with the other pillars, particularly control and precision. The deliberate engagement of the mind ensures that movements are executed with precision, and the sustained focus contributes to the overall control of the body. The combination of concentration, control, and precision results in a Wall Pilates practice that goes beyond the superficial, creating a profound transformation in both physical and mental realms.

The meditative quality of concentration in Wall Pilates distinguishes it from more conventional forms of exercise. As you tune into the subtleties of your movements, you embark on a journey of self-discovery. This approach extends to breath awareness, with each inhalation and exhalation serving as a rhythm for movement, creating a harmonious integration of breath and motion. The ability to focus on the present moment developed through Pilates concentration becomes a valuable asset for managing stress and maintaining a sense of calm amidst life's challenges as you forge into and beyond your senior years.

Flow

The flow principle in Wall Pilates refers to the seamless and continuous transition between movements, creating a harmonious and rhythmic sequence. This dynamic quality contributes to the practice's overall effectiveness and enhances physical and mental benefits.

In Wall Pilates, flow is about more than just moving from one exercise to the next. It involves a smooth and controlled progression through each phase of a workout. While performing the exercises, you're encouraged to maintain a constant and deliberate flow, ensuring that one movement seamlessly leads into the next.

The flow principle is closely connected to breath, as the rhythm of breath becomes a guiding force for movement. Inhales and exhales are synchronized with the various phases of an exercise, creating a natural ebb and flow that supports the practice's physical and mental aspects.

This dynamic flow is particularly evident in the way Wall Pilates exercises are often linked together in a series. The seamless transition between exercises that the Wall allows challenges you to maintain control and precision, reinforcing the interconnected nature of Wall Pilates movements.

The Pillars of Power in Wall Pilates, such as breathing correctly, control, centering, precision, concentration, and flow, form the foundation of this transformative exercise system. Together, they create a comprehensive foundation beyond physical fitness and delve into mental discipline, mindfulness, and holistic well-being. Mastering these pillars will build strength, flexibility, and endurance and cultivate a profound connection between mind and body.

Chapter 3:
Warm Up & Cool Down

Preparation Tips

If you've ever tried to exercise without warming up, you're probably already aware of the aches, pains and possible injuries that can ensue. Warming up is therefore a *must,* not just in your senior years, but at any stage of life. Here are some essential things to consider when warming up for Wall Pilates exercises:

Safety

Safety is paramount in any exercise routine. The warm-up phase is crucial for preparing your body for the specific demands of Wall Pilates exercises to minimize the risk of injury and promote an effective and enjoyable workout. Key safety considerations to keep in mind include:

1. Physical Readiness

Before engaging in Wall Pilates, assess your physical readiness. If you have any pre-existing health conditions, injuries, or concerns, it is essential to consult with a healthcare professional or a qualified Pilates instructor. This step ensures that you embark on Wall Pilates with a clear understanding of potential limitations and the necessary modifications for your situation.

2. Proper Form Emphasis

Establishing good form sets the foundation for the entire workout, reducing the risk of strain or injury. Whether performing dynamic stretches or engaging with the wall for resistance, consider alignment and controlled movements carefully. This emphasis on proper form extends throughout the warm-up and into the main Wall Pilates routine.

3. Gradual Progression

Progress through your workout routine gradually. This may sound easier said than done, but if you're warmed up, it does become a lot simpler. Listen to your body and adjust the intensity of your workout based on how you feel.

4. Joint Protection with Controlled Movements

Prioritize joint protection by incorporating controlled movements into your workout. Wall Pilates involves various motions. Ensuring that these movements are deliberate and controlled helps protect your joints. Focus on controlled leg lifts, gentle twists, and dynamic stretches that promote joint mobility without placing unnecessary stress on them.

5. Warm-Up Duration

Adequate warm-up duration is crucial for preparing your muscles and joints for the upcoming Wall Pilates exercises. Allocate sufficient time for your warm-up, typically around 5-7 minutes, to allow for gradual increases in heart rate, blood flow, and body temperature and optimize your body's readiness for more intense movements.

6. Listen to Your Body

Pay close attention to how your body responds throughout the exercises. If you experience any pain, discomfort, or unusual sensations, be responsive to these signals, don't just ignore them, chalking them up to age. Modify movements or stop if necessary. Exercises should not cause pain; they should gently prepare your body for the challenges ahead.

7. Appropriate Attire and Footwear

Wear comfortable and appropriate attire for Wall Pilates. Clothing should allow for a full range of motion without restricting movement. Choose supportive athletic footwear or non-slip socks, especially if your routine involves standing exercises. Proper footwear enhances stability and protects your feet during dynamic movements.

Space Requirements

Creating a suitable and safe space is crucial for effectively executing Wall Pilates exercises. The right environment ensures ample room for movement, reduces the risk of injury, and enhances the overall experience of your warm-up routine. Some things to think about when choosing the best place to practice Wall Pilates:

1. Clearance Around the Wall

Ensure sufficient clearance around the wall where you'll perform Wall Pilates exercises. Remove any obstacles or furniture that may impede your movements. This clear space allows you to engage in a full range of motion without the risk of bumping into objects, providing a safe and unobstructed practice area.

2. Mat or Exercise Surface

Place a non-slip mat or exercise surface on the floor to provide a comfortable and stable foundation for your exercises, especially if you engage in floor-based movements. The mat enhances safety by preventing slips and supports exercises involving sitting or lying during the workout.

3. Ample Room for Arm and Leg Movements

Wall Pilates exercises often involve arm and leg movements in a standing position and on the mat. You won't be flailing about, but you need enough space to fully extend your arms and legs. Ensure ample room for dynamic stretches, arm circles, leg swings, and controlled leg lifts. Having sufficient space allows for unrestricted movements and a more enjoyable experience.

4. Proximity to a Wall

Position yourself near a stable wall. The wall will serve as a support and resistance during the warm-up and workout. This may sound a bit like pointing out the obvious, but you should check that the wall is free from any sharp objects or protrusions that could pose a safety hazard. Proximity to the wall is essential for exercises that involve leaning, pressing, or utilizing the wall for resistance. If there is a wall hanging or picture frame above the area where you are exercising, remove it for safety.

5. Good Lighting and Ventilation

Optimal lighting is essential for safety and focus during the workout routine. Ensure that the space is well-lit, either with natural or artificial light. Proper lighting reduces the risk of tripping or missteps. Additionally, good ventilation promotes a comfortable workout environment as your body temperature increases while exercising.

The Warm-Up

An effective warm-up for Wall Pilates should encompass various preparation techniques that gradually engage the muscles and increase the heart rate. The goal is to prepare the body and mind for the specific demands of Wall Pilates exercises.

1. Cardiovascular Activation - Begin with light cardiovascular exercises to elevate the heart rate. The aim is to increase blood flow, warm the muscles, and enhance overall circulation.

2. Joint Mobilization - Perform gentle joint mobilization exercises to increase mobility and lubricate the joints. Focus on wrists, ankles, shoulders, and hips.

3. Dynamic Stretching - Incorporate dynamic stretches to enhance flexibility and improve range of motion. Dynamic stretching prepares the muscles for more active movements and helps prevent injury.

4. Pilates-Specific Movements - Integrate Pilates inspired movements into your warm-up. Include standing roll-downs, controlled leg lifts, and gentle spinal twists. These movements engage the core and prepare the body for the specific demands of Wall Pilates.

5. Mindful Visualization - Close your eyes and visualize yourself moving through Wall Pilates exercises with precision and control. Envision your core's engagement, the wall's support, and the fluidity of your movements. Visualization primes the mind for the upcoming workout.

Warm-up routines you can try for Wall Pilates include:

Breathing	Put your hands above your waist on your rib cage. Breath in through your nose, engaging your core. Exhale while tightening your core. Repeat 4 times.
Arm Raises	In a standing position bring your arms up and down while inhaling (arms up) and exhaling (arms down) Repeat 6 times.
Shoulder Rolls	Roll both shoulders forward in a circular motion. Repeat 10 times forward and 10 times backward.
Wrist and Ankle Rotations	Rotate both wrists gently 10 times on each direction. Do the same with your ankles one at the time.
Arm Stretches	Raise your arms straight out in front of you with fingers pointing upward. Then move your arms straight out to the sides, then back to center. Repeat 4 times.
Side Reach	While standing, exhale as you reach up over your head with your right arm, bending to the left. Exhale, then return to center. Repeat other side. (6 times total)
Knee Raises	While standing with hands on your waist, lift one knee to a ninety-degree angle. Bring your leg back down and lift 5 more 6 times. Switch legs and repeat twice.
Ankle Raises	Turn to your side and put one arm against the wall, raise your ankles up and down 10 times.

Breathing

The synchronization of breath with movement is a fundamental principle that extends throughout the Wall Pilates practice, including the warm-up and cool-down phase. Conscious and controlled breathing is pivotal in enhancing the mind-body connection, promoting relaxation, and preparing the body for the specific demands of Wall Pilates exercises. You can incorporate breathing throughout your exercise routine.

1. Diaphragmatic Breathing

Emphasize diaphragmatic breathing, also known as deep belly breathing. Inhale deeply and slowly through the nose, allowing the breath to expand the ribcage and fill the lungs. Exhale through the mouth, drawing the navel toward the spine. This rhythmic breathing pattern promotes relaxation and engages the core.

2. Coordination with Movements

Coordinate your breath with each movement during the exercise routine. For example, inhale during the initial phase of a stretch or move and exhale during the release or return phase. This coordination enhances control and focus.

3. Breath as a Guide

Allow your breath to serve as a guide for the pace and rhythm of each exercise. A steady and controlled breath pattern supports precision and intentional movements required in Wall Pilates. Use your breath as a tool to enhance concentration.

4. Mindful Breath Awareness

Take moments during the practice to cultivate mindful breath awareness. Close your eyes, tune into the sensation of your breath, and bring your attention to the present moment. This conscious awareness fosters a deeper connection between your breath, body, and the support of the wall.

5. Adapt Breathing to Movements

Adapt your breathing pattern to the various Wall Pilates movements. For dynamic stretches, you might coordinate your breath with the rhythm of the movement. During static stretches, maintain a steady and relaxed breath to promote a sense of ease and openness.

6. Breath Integration with Core Engagement

The warm-up phase is an opportune time to integrate breath awareness with core engagement. As you engage in controlled movements against the wall or perform gentle stretches, synchronize your breath with activating your core muscles.

7. Relaxation and Stress Reduction

Controlled breathing during the exercise routine contributes to relaxation and stress reduction. The deliberate inhalation and exhalation patterns activate the parasympathetic nervous system, promoting a state of calmness. This breathing aspect benefits physical preparation and creates a conducive mental and emotional environment for the Wall Pilates session.

Cooling Down

Proper cooling is as crucial as the warm-up in completing a Wall Pilates session. It aids in recovery, flexibility, and relaxation. Cooling down allows the body to gradually return to a resting state reducing the heartrate and minimizing post-workout stiffness and soreness. Some cool-down routines you can try for Wall Pilates include:

Neck Stretch	While standing, tilt your head to once side. Bring it back to center and tilt it to the other side. Repeat 4 times
Back Stretch	Raise your arms towards the ceiling interlocking your fingers. Feel the stretch in your arms and back. Then lower your arms back down. Repeat 3 times.
Hamstring Stretch	Leaning your back against the wall with legs slightly wider than your hips, bend forward and grab your ankles. Let your head hang. Hold 15 seconds then return back to up position. Repeat 3 times.
Hip Flexor Stretch	Laying face up on your mat, bring your knees to your chest, wrap your arms around them and rock your body from side to side 4 times.
Arm Raises	In a standing position bring your arms up and down while inhaling (arms up) and exhaling (arms down) Repeat 6 times.

Chapter 4:
Exercise Instructions

Wall Calf Stretch

The Wall Calf Stretch is a stretching exercise that targets the calf muscles. The stretch promotes the length of your two calf muscles, the soleus, which is down toward the Achilles tendon, and the gastrocnemius, the belly of the calf. This exercise can help prevent shin splints, plantar fasciitis, and calf strains.

- **Starting Position**: Stand facing the wall with your hands pressed against it and toes about one foot from the wall. Your arms should remain straight and your palms flat against the wall.
- **Movement**: Step one foot back, keeping the heel on the ground, and press into the wall.
- **End Position**: Feel the stretch in your calf. Hold for 5 seconds and switch sides. Repeat each side 4 times.

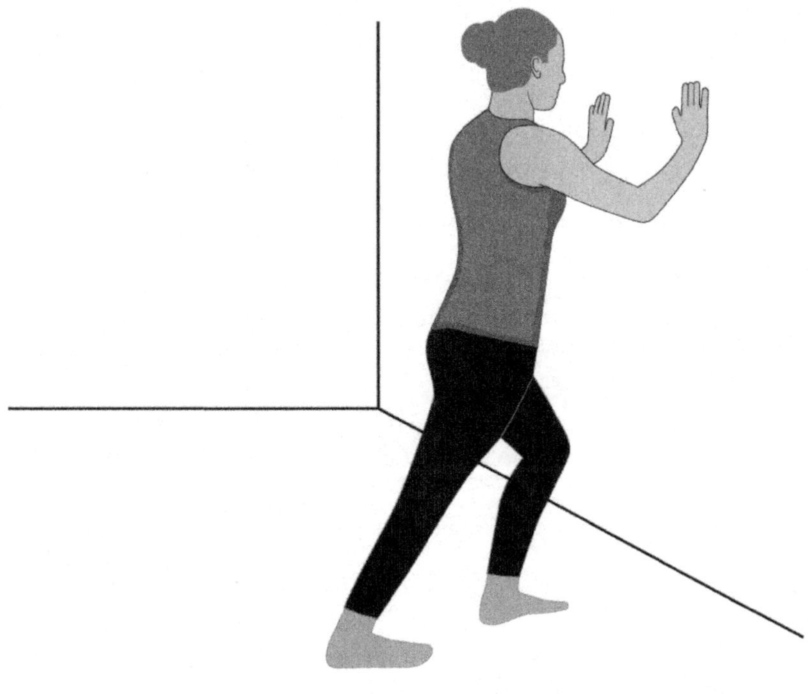

WALL CALF STRETCH

Wall Chest Stretch

The Wall Chest Stretch is a therapeutic and flexible exercise that involves opening the chest and shoulders. This stretch aims to counteract the effects of poor posture, sedentary activities, or tightness in the chest muscles by lengthening the muscles across the chest and shoulders.

- **Starting Position**: Face the wall, then outstretch your left arm placing your palm on the wall.
- **Movement**: Slowly rotate your torso to the right and feel the stretch in your chest and left shoulder. Keep your palm pressed against the wall. Hold 15 seconds.
- **End Position**: Breathe out when deepening the stretch. Repeat on both sides for a total of 3 times.

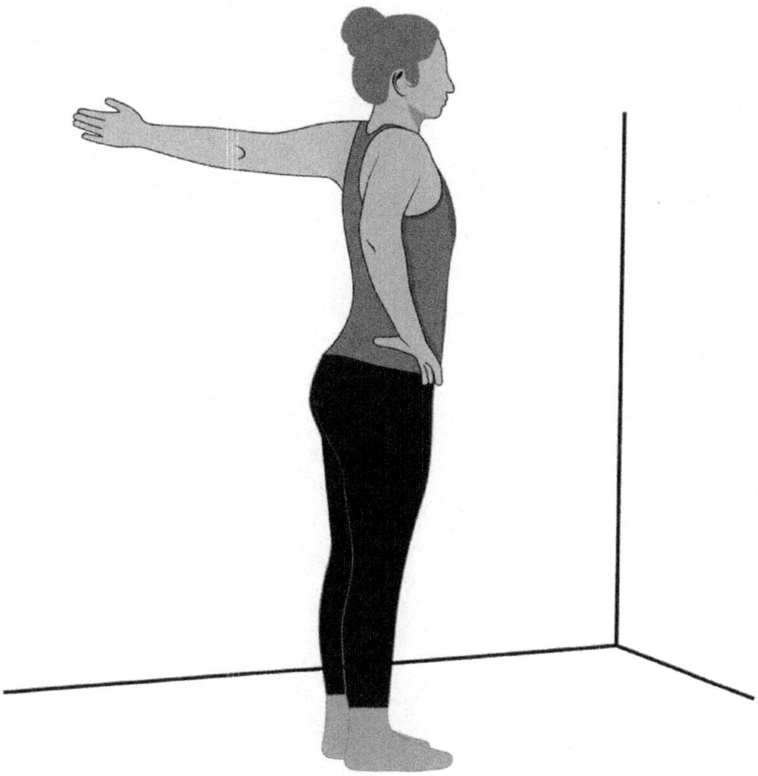

WALL CHEST STRETCH

Wall Arm Circles

Wall Arm Circles are a gentle, low-impact exercise designed to improve shoulder mobility, flexibility, and overall upper body function. This exercise involves making circular motions with the arms while leaning against a wall for support. Wall Arm Circles provide a safe and effective way to enhance the range of motion in the shoulder joints.

- **Starting Position:** Stand with your back against the wall and arms extended to the sides.
- **Movement**: Begin by making small circular motions moving both arms simultaneously clockwise. Focus on control.
- **End Position**: Repeat the circular motions for 30 seconds going clockwise, then rest for 15 seconds. Repeat again counterclockwise.

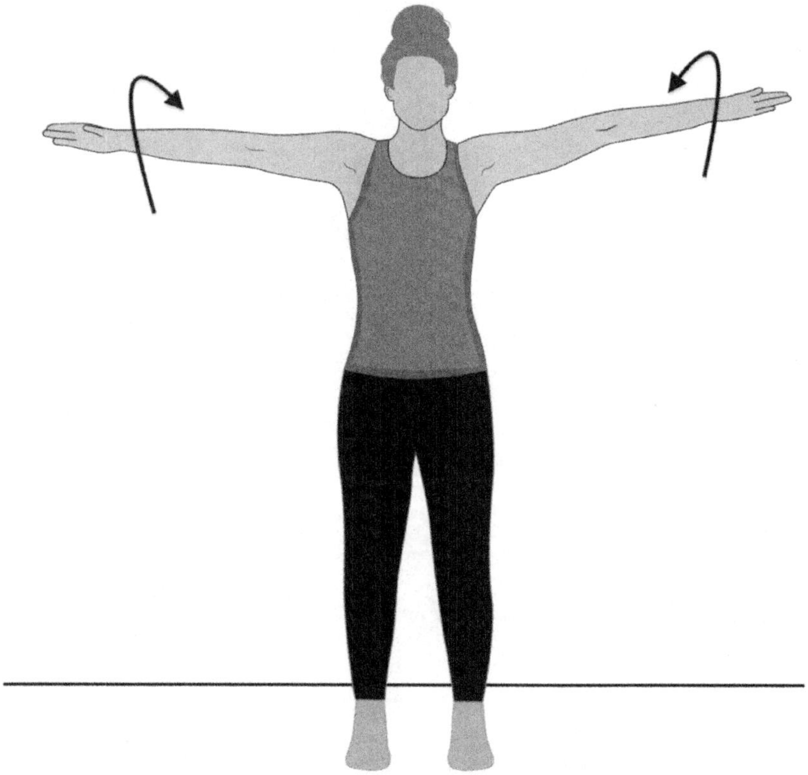

WALL ARM CIRCLES

Wall Shoulder Blade Squeeze

The Wall Shoulder Blade Squeeze is a targeted exercise that involves retracting and squeezing the shoulder blades together while standing with the back against a wall. This movement focuses on strengthening the muscles between the shoulder blades, promoting improved posture and shoulder stability.

- **Starting Position**: Stand with your back against the wall and arms extended to the sides in a W position. Keep your feet hip-width apart and ensure the back of your head, shoulders, and hips contact the wall.
- **Movement**: Squeeze your shoulder blades together, bringing your arms toward each other along the wall.
- **End Position**: Hold for a moment and release. Repeat for 2 sets of 10 repetitions.

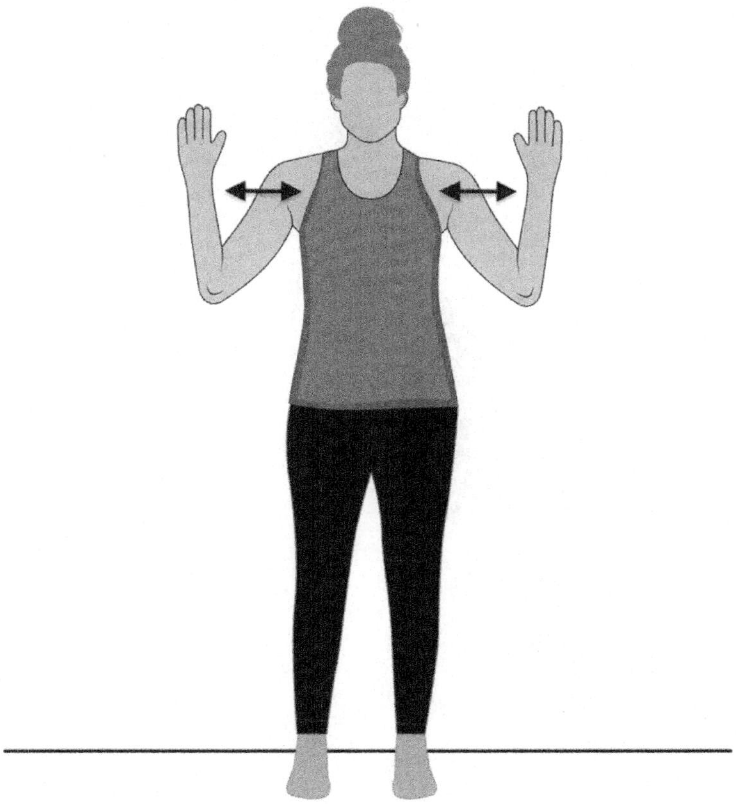

WALL SHOULDER BLADE SQUEEZE

Wall Plank

The Wall Plank is a modified variation of the traditional plank exercise, making it a suitable option for seniors concerned about performing a conventional plank on the floor.

- **Starting Position**: Stand facing the wall at arm's length, with your feet hip-width apart. Place your forearms against the wall shoulder-width apart with your elbows at a 90-degree angle.
- **Movement**: Step your feet back once more, keeping them hip-apart and engaging the core.
- **End Position**: Hold for 20 seconds and repeat 3 more times.

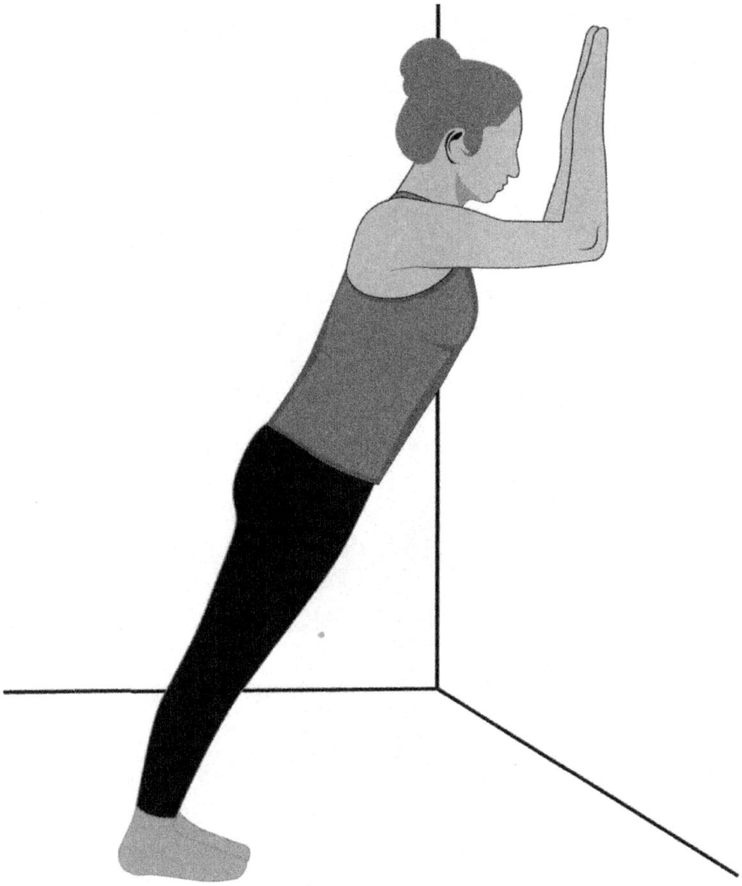

WALL PLANK

Wall Side Bend

The wall-assisted side bend is designed to stretch and strengthen the muscles along the sides of the torso. The side bend engages the core and promotes lateral flexibility.

- **Starting Position**: Stand with your side facing the wall, place the hand closest to the wall against it.
- **Movement**: Inhale as you reach the free arm overhead, extending through the side of the body. Exhale as you bend the upper body sideways.
- **End Position**: Hold the stretched position momentarily and inhale as you return to the starting position. Perform 2 sets of 10 reps on each side.

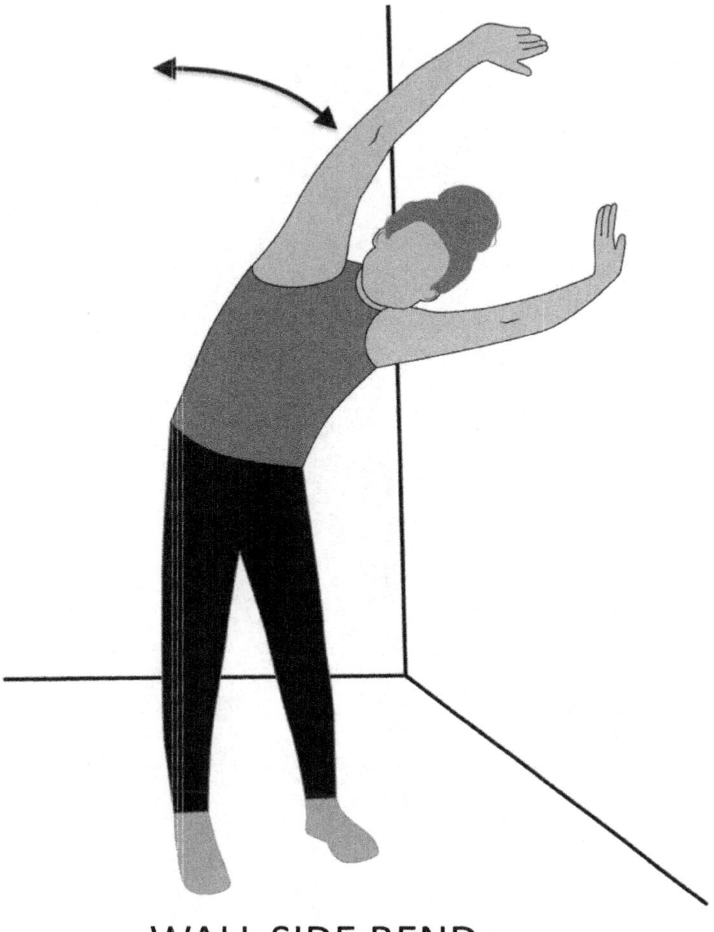

WALL SIDE BEND

Standing Wall Twist

This is a gentle and effective exercise that improves rotational flexibility in the spine. It is performed with the support of a wall to provide stability and promote proper alignment. It targets the muscles of the torso and enhances mobility in the upper body.

- **Starting Position**: Stand with your back pressed against the wall and feet hip-width apart.
- **Movement**: Keep your feet planted and twist your torso to one side, bringing your hands together on the wall. Hold for a moment, feeling a gentle stretch.
- **End Position**: Now move your hands and torso together to your other side, and hold. Repeat this motion 10 times.

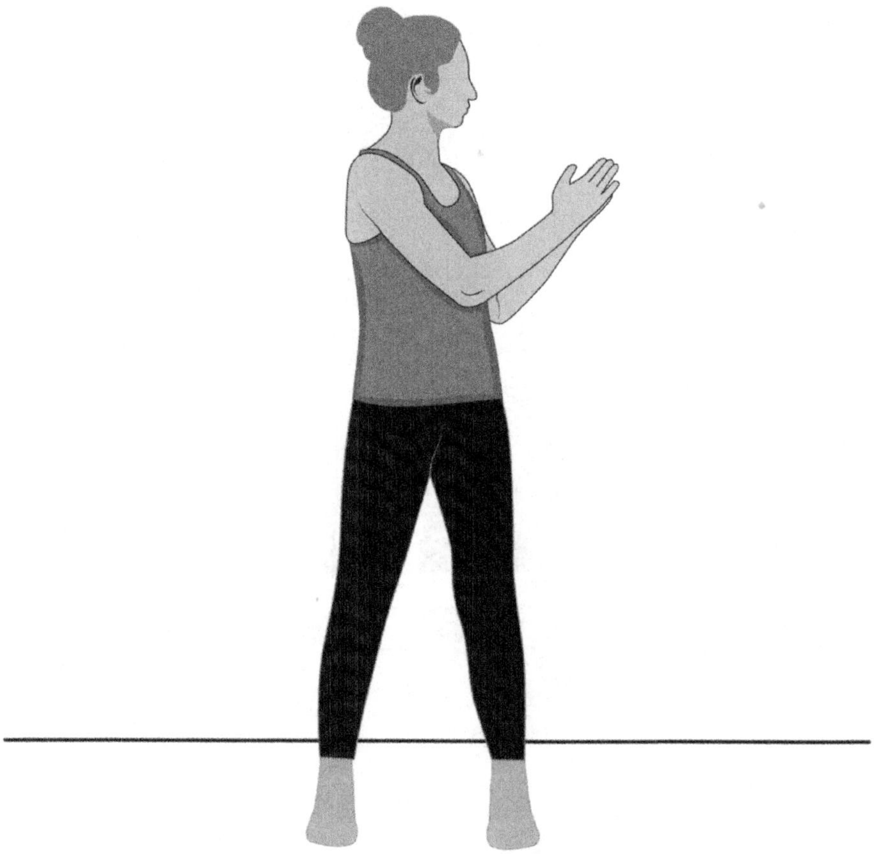

STANDING WALL TWIST

Wall Heel Raises

Wall-assisted heel raises target the calf muscles, specifically the gastrocnemius and soleus. A wall for support provides stability, making it a safe and effective way for seniors who need balance assistance to work on calf strength and ankle flexibility.

- **Starting Position**: Place your hands lightly on the wall at shoulder height and feet hip-width apart.
- **Movement**: Rise onto your toes, lifting your heels off the ground by pressing through the balls of your feet.
- **End Position**: Lower your heels back down and repeat for 2 sets of 10 while maintaining a controlled pace.

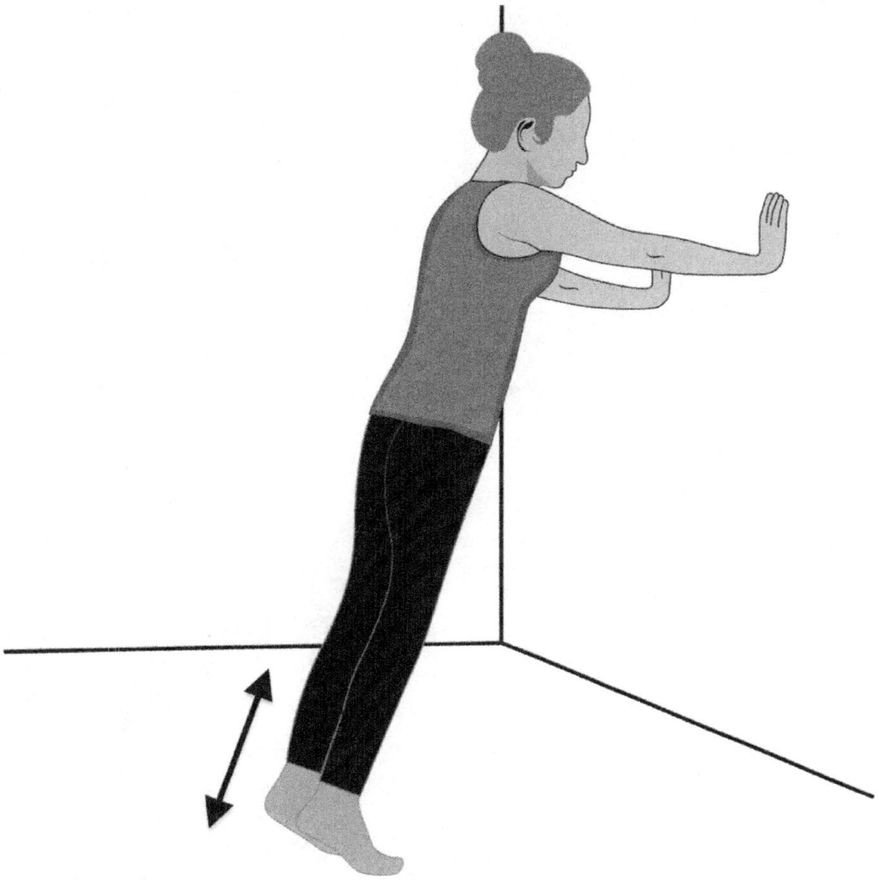

WALL HEEL RAISES

Wall Leg Raises

The Wall-Assisted Leg Raises targets your glutes, hamstrings, and lower back. Ensure your hips stay level throughout the movement. Keep shoulders relaxed and away from your ears.

- **Starting Position**: With outstretched arms, place both palms of your hands on the wall at shoulder height. Take one more step back keeping your hands on the wall.
- **Movement**: Raise one leg straight back to a comfortable height, ensuring you feel the engagement in the hamstring and hip.
- **End Position**: Perform 10 repetitions, then lower the leg and switch to the other leg. Repeat 2 sets in total.

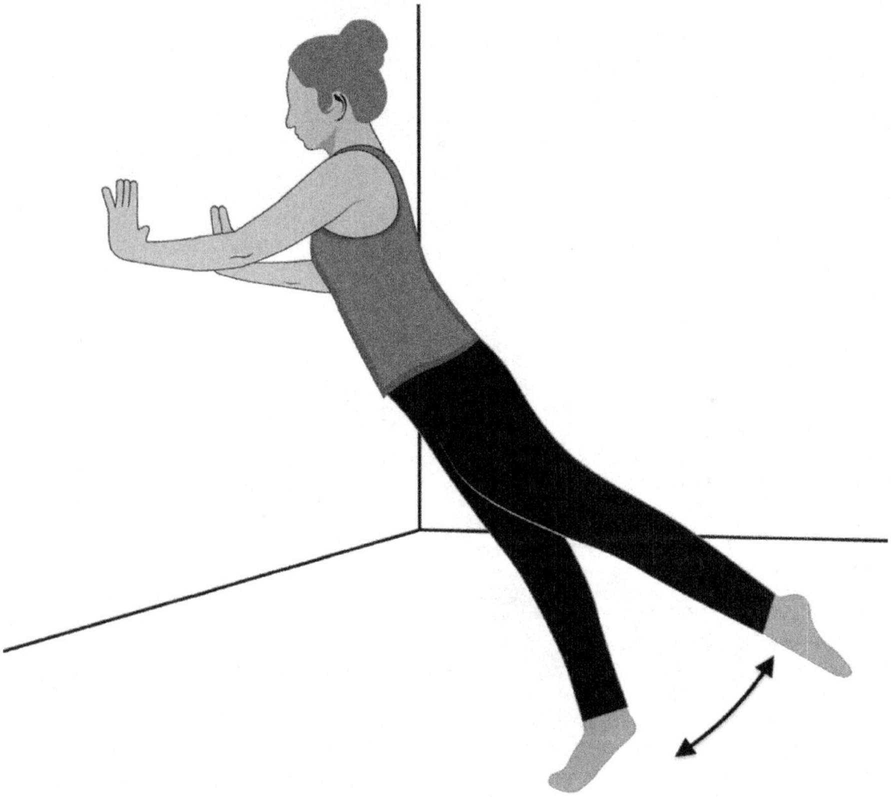

WALL LEG RAISES

Wall Marching

Wall marching is a simple yet effective exercise involving lifting your knees alternately. It combines elements of cardiovascular activity with strength training, engaging multiple muscle groups in the lower body and core.

- **Starting Position**: Stand with your back against a wall, ensuring your entire back is in contact with the wall. Maintain an upright posture with your shoulders relaxed and your head aligned with your spine.
- **Movement**: Lift one knee toward your chest while keeping the other foot on the ground as if marching.
- **End Position**: March in a controlled motion. Aim for 3 sets, marching 30 seconds per set. Rest between sets.

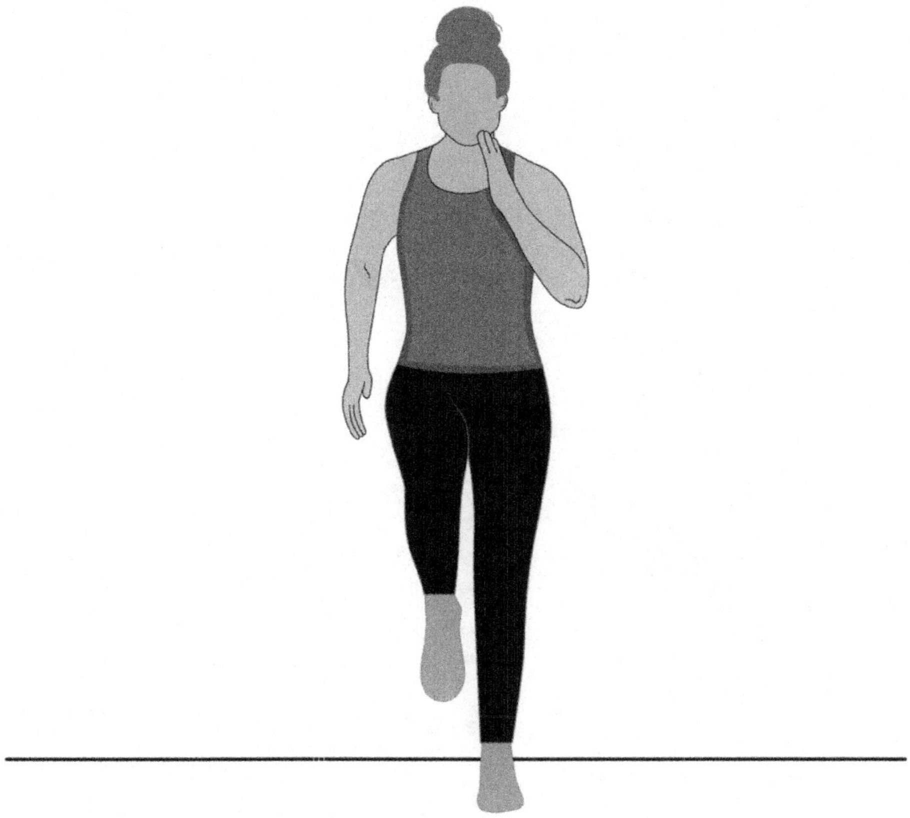

WALL MARCHING

Wall Side Leg Lifts

Wall-assisted side leg lifts are an exercise that targets the muscles of the outer thighs (abductors) and hips. This variation involves using a wall for support and stability, making it an accessible and effective way to work on hip strength and leg mobility. The movement is gentle on the joints and still provides effective muscle engagement.

- **Starting Position**: Stand with your side facing the wall and hands pressed against it.
- **Movement**: Lift one leg to the side, engaging your outer thigh. Raise your leg to a comfortable height, ensuring you feel the engagement in the thigh and hip.
- **End Position**: Lower the leg and repeat on the other side. Perform 2 sets of 10 repetitions on each side.

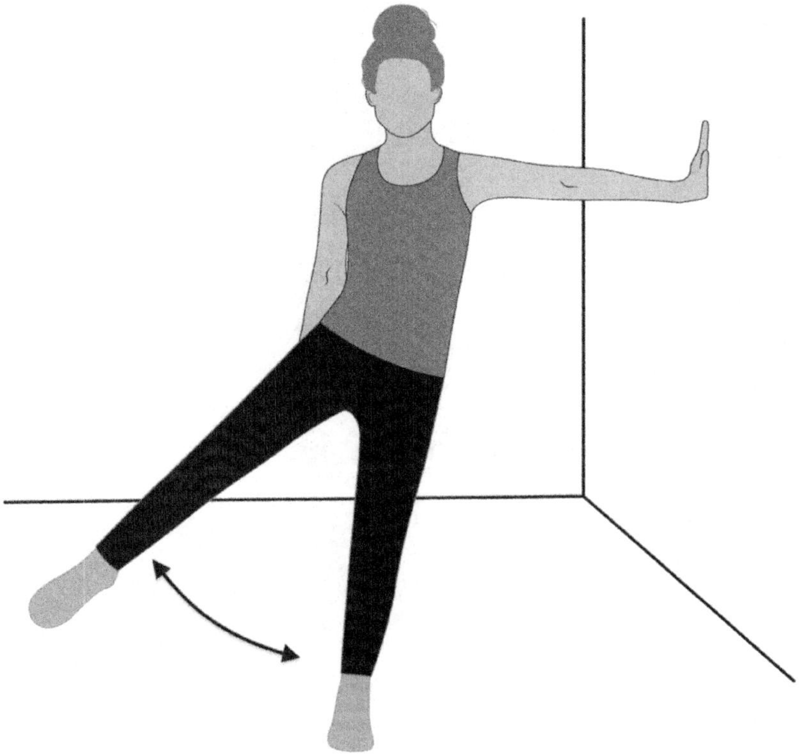

WALL SIDE LEG LIFTS

Wall Push Ups

Wall push-ups are designed to be more accessible, especially for seniors with limited upper body strength. This variation provides a gentler introduction to upper body strengthening. Wall push-ups are gentle on the wrists and shoulders, making them suitable for seniors.

- **Starting Position**: Stand facing the wall, about arm's length away. Place your hands on the wall at shoulder height, slightly wider than shoulder width apart.
- **Movement**: Keep your body straight from head to heels and inhale as you bend your elbows, lowering your chest toward the wall.
- **End Position**: Exhale as you push away from the wall, straightening your arms. Start with 2 sets of 10 repetitions.

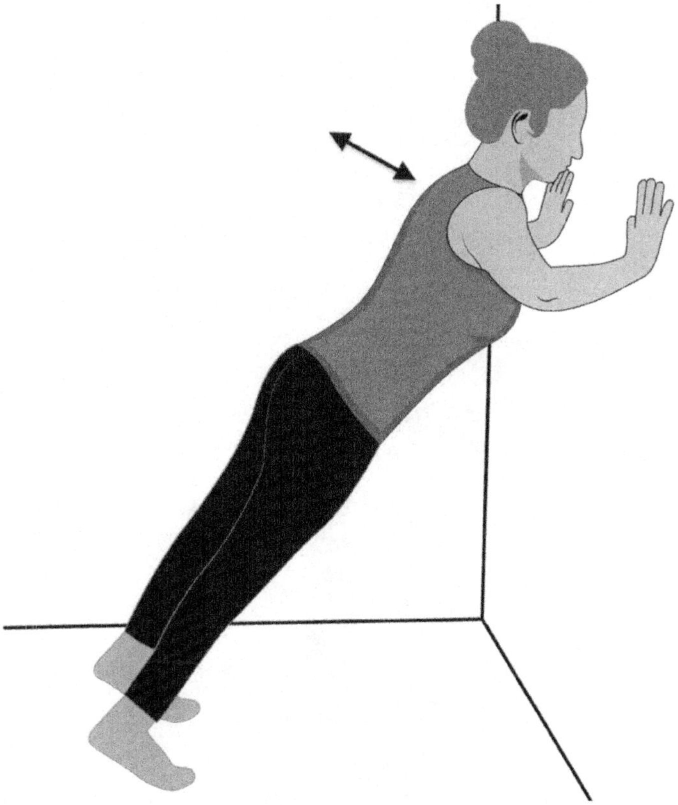

WALL PUSH UPS

Wall Roll Down

The Wall Roll Down is a modified version of the traditional Pilates roll-down exercise, adapted to be performed with the support of a wall. It focuses on improving flexibility in the spine and engaging the core muscles.

- **Starting Position**: Stand with your back against the wall and feet hip-width apart. Your feet should be a few inches away from the wall.
- **Movement**: Inhale deeply, then exhale as you initiate the roll down by tucking your chin to your chest and gently lowering your head toward your chest. Go down as far as you can with your core engaged.
- **End Position**: Inhale at the bottom, then roll back up to the starting position as you exhale. Perform 2 sets of 6 repetitions.

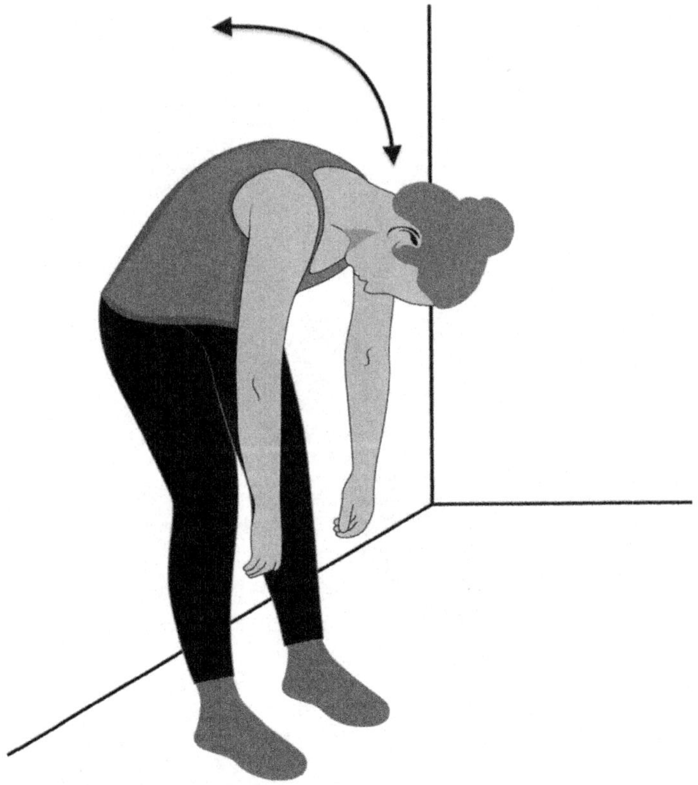

WALL ROLL DOWNS

Wall Sit

The wall sit is an effective exercise for building endurance and lower body strength. It's an isometric exercise to help you target your hamstrings, quadriceps, glutes, and core muscles. The simple movements of this exercise can increase muscle tone and enhance stability.

- **Starting Position**: Stand with your back against the wall and feet hip-width apart, positioned around two feet away from the wall. The head, shoulders, and lower back should be in contact with the wall.
- **Movement**: Slide your back down the wall slowly, bending your knees until they reach a 90-degree angle.
- **End Position**: Hold the seated position engaging your thigh muscles. Aim for 3 sets of 15 seconds each.

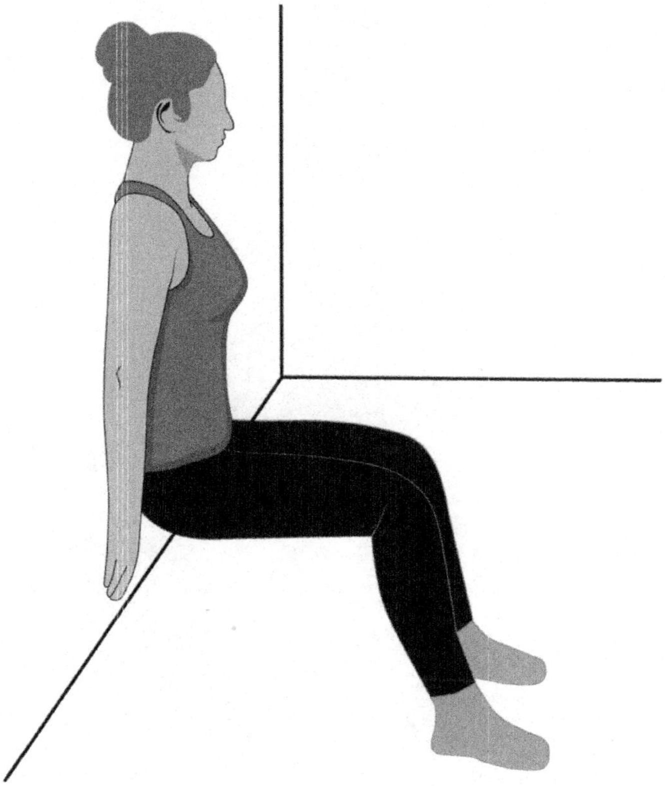

WALL SIT

Leg Press against the Wall

The leg press against the wall is a lower body exercise that engages the muscles of the legs, particularly the quadriceps, hamstrings, and glutes. This exercise is performed against a wall, providing resistance for the legs while incorporating elements of stability and control.

- **Starting Position**: Stand with your back against the wall and walk your feet out slightly from the wall.
- **Movement**: Keep your back and head against the wall, sliding your back down the wall just a few inches until your knees are slightly bent.
- **End Position**: Hold momentarily, then push through your feet to slide back up the wall to the starting position. Perform 2 sets of 8 repetitions.

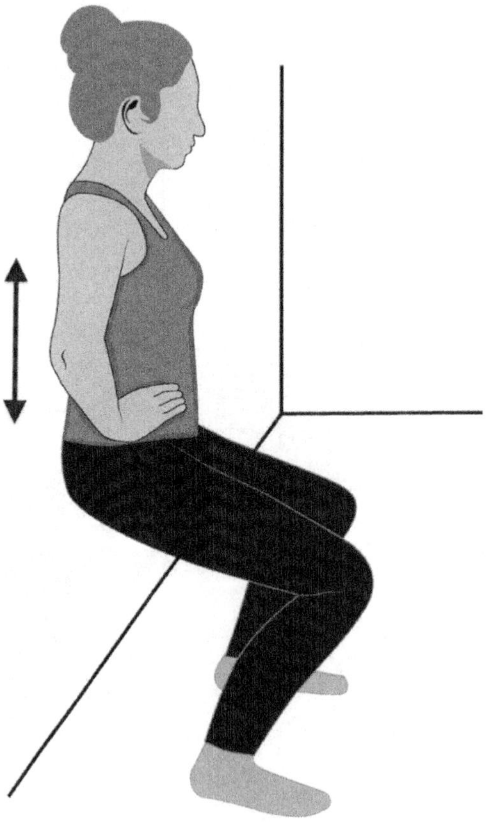

LEG PRESS AGAINST THE WALL

Wall Lunges

Wall lunges are a modified version of the traditional lunge exercise, using a wall for support and stability. This variation is particularly beneficial for seniors needing additional assistance with balance.

- **Starting Position**: Stand with one side of your body parallel to the wall bracing with your hand for extra support.
- **Movement**: Take a large step back with the outside leg and drop into the lunge position. Maintain a straight line up from your knee to your hip to your shoulder.
- **End Position**: Focus on slowly lowering yourself just a few inches and pushing yourself back up – for a total of 8 times. Repeat with the opposite leg. Perform 2 sets.

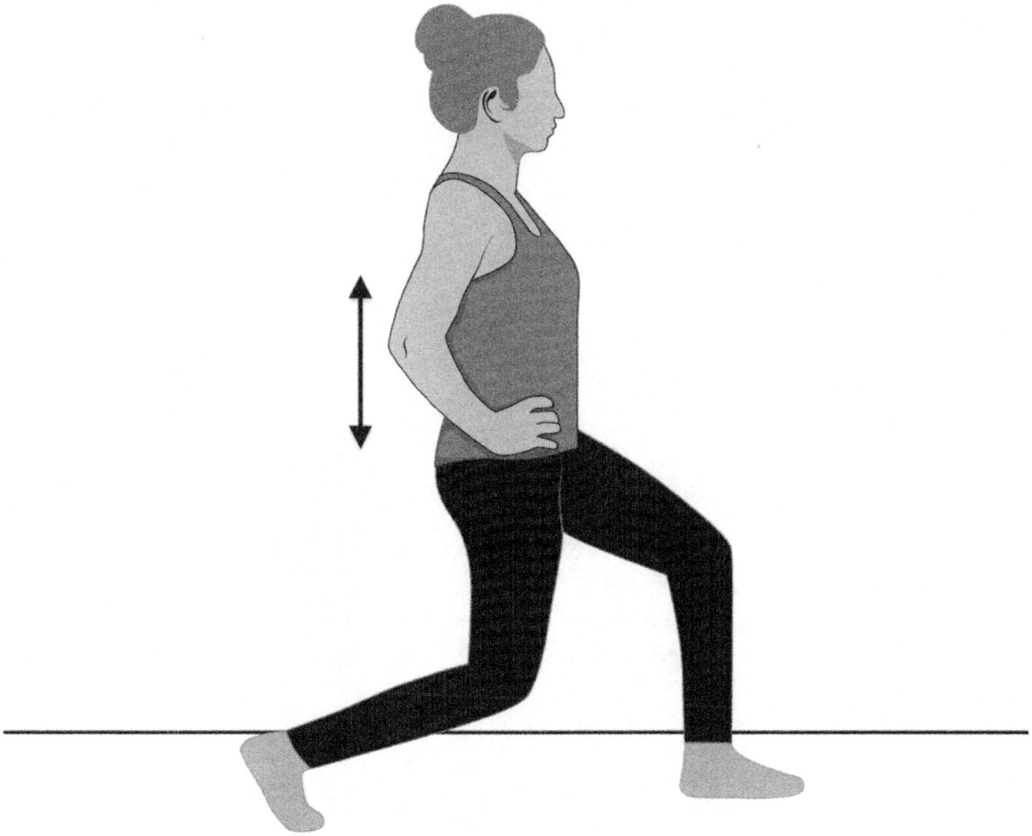

WALL LUNGES

Wall Hip Flexor Stretch

This is a dynamic stretching exercise targeting hip flexors and quadriceps muscles. This stretch is performed with the support of a wall to provide stability and facilitate proper alignment during the movement. It is an effective way to improve flexibility, reduce muscle tightness, and enhance the range of motion in the hip region.

- **Starting Position**: Kneel in front of a wall facing away.
- **Movement**: Keeping your left knee on the floor, raise your left foot behind you and rest it against the wall. Step your right leg out with the foot flat on the floor and the knee bent, thigh parallel to the floor.
- **End Position**: Hold the stretch for 15 seconds on each leg and repeat 2 times. Use a cushion under knee for comfort.

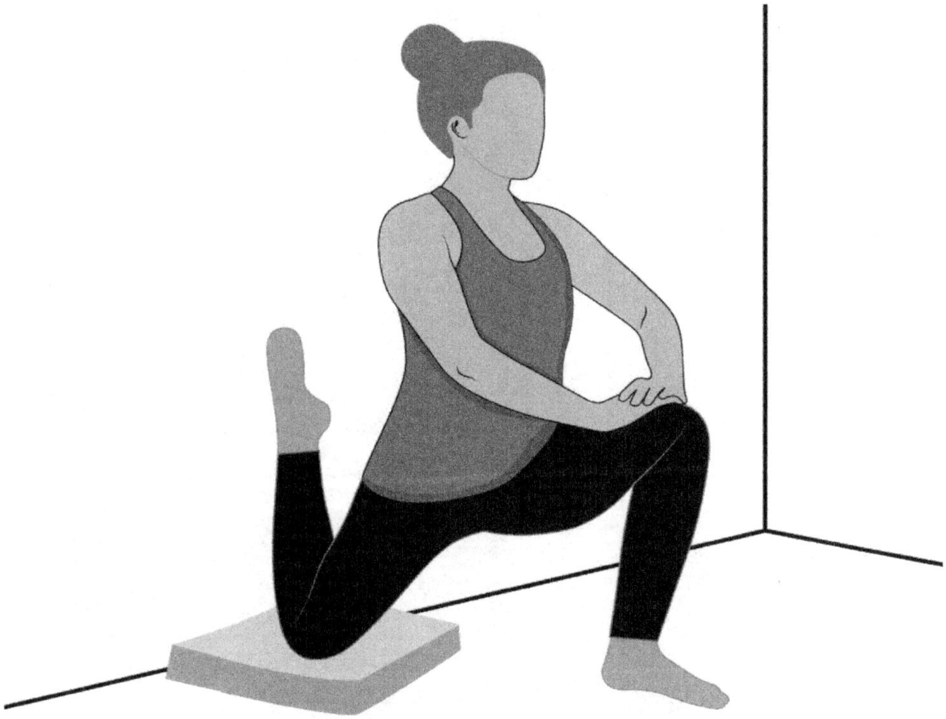

WALL HIP FLEXOR STRETCH

Seated Leg Lifts

Seated leg lifts are a Pilates exercise designed to target and strengthen the core, hips, and thigh muscles. This variation adds an extra element of stability by using the support of a wall, making it suitable for seniors of varying fitness levels, and those with limited mobility.

- **Starting Position**: Sit on the floor, back against the wall and your legs extended in front of you. Place your hands on the floor beside your hips for support.
- **Movement**: Lift one leg off the floor, keeping it straight, and hold for a moment.
- **End Position**: Lower the leg back down with control. Perform 2 sets of 10 repetitions for each leg.

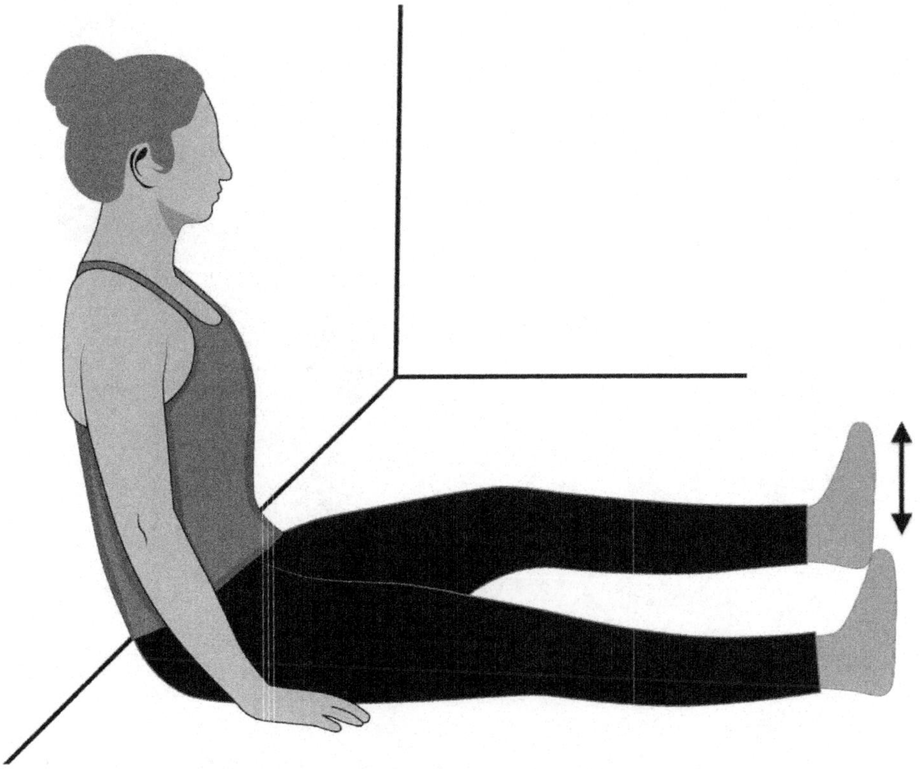

SEATED LEG LIFTS

Bent Leg Wall Hundred

The Bent Leg Wall Hundred is a modification of the classical "Hundred." This variation is adapted to be performed against a wall, providing support and stability. This targets the core muscles, promotes abdominal strength, and enhances overall endurance.

- **Starting Position**: Lie on your back with your feet flat against the wall and knees bent. Extend your arms straight out in front but lifted off the floor.
- **Movement**: Lift your head and shoulders off the mat, tightening your core muscles, and quickly pump your arms up and down. Inhale for five arm pumps and exhale for five arm pumps, continuing the pattern.
- **End Position**: Pump your arms for 20 seconds. Take a 15 second rest and do 2 more sets.

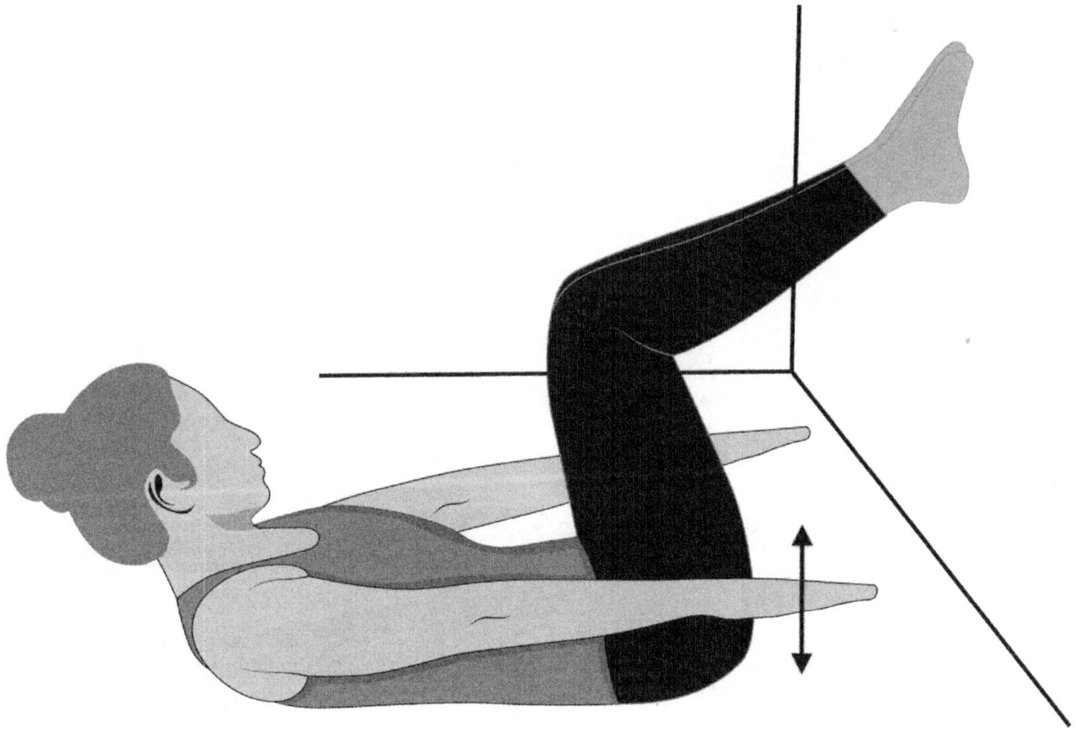

BENT LEG WALL HUNDRED

Wall Heel Slides

Wall-assisted heel slides combine gentle leg movements with the support of a wall. This exercise is designed to improve flexibility, mobility, and strength in the lower body, targeting the muscles of the thighs and hamstrings.

- **Starting Position**: Start by lying on your back with your butt close to (or touching) the wall, knees bent, and feet resting on the wall.
- **Movement**: Straighten both legs by sliding your feet up the wall. Hold the position for a few seconds.
- **End Position**: Bend your right knee and slide your foot down the wall as shown in the illustration. Do 2 sets of 8 repetitions for each leg.

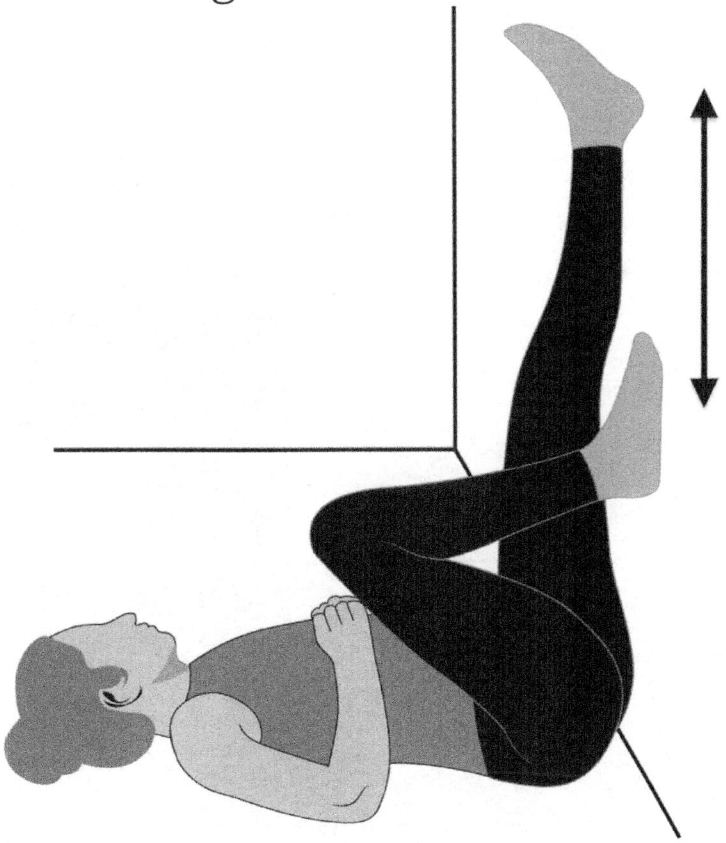

WALL HEEL SLIDES

Wall Hip Bridge

The wall hip bridge is a modified version of the traditional hip bridge exercise, designed to be a more accessible lower-body workout for seniors or individuals with mobility concerns. This exercise targets the lower back muscles, buttocks, and hamstrings while providing support and stability.

- **Starting Position**: Lie down on your back with your feet flat on the wall, hip-width apart. Place your arms by your sides with your palms facing down.
- **Movement**: Press through your heels and engage your glutes to lift your hips toward the ceiling while inhaling.
- **End Position**: Hold the lifted position for a moment and lower your hips back down to the floor in a controlled manner while exhaling. Perform 2 sets of 8 of repetitions.

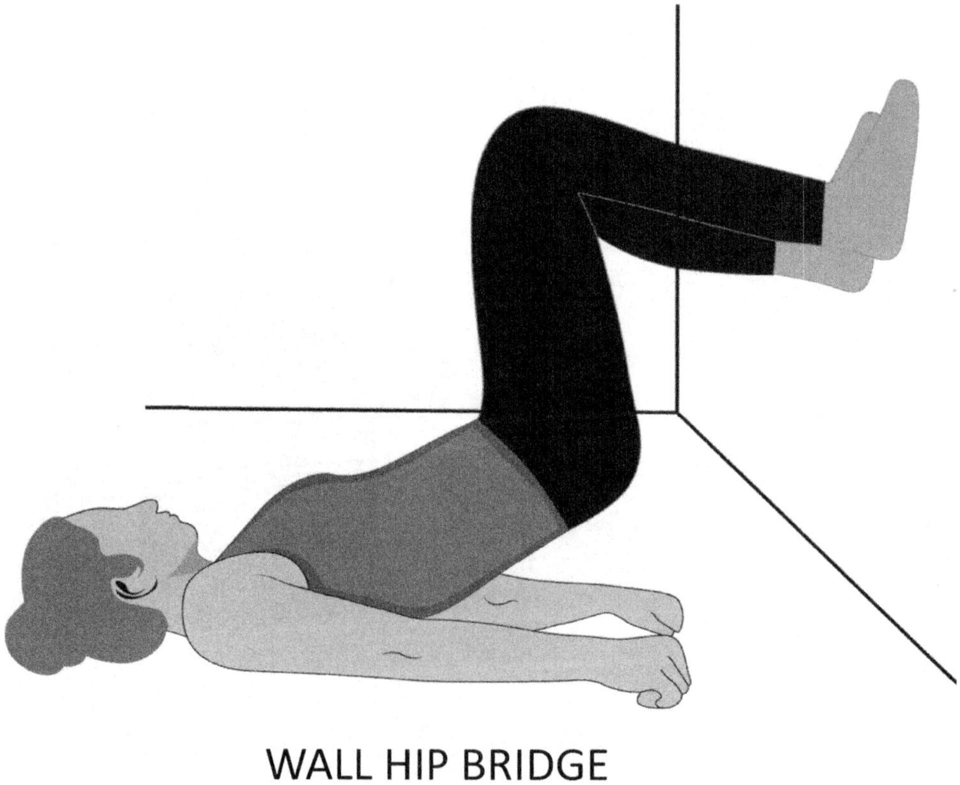

WALL HIP BRIDGE

Wall Bridge with Leg Lift

This combines the traditional bridge position with the added challenge of lifting one leg toward the ceiling. It promotes strength, stability, and flexibility and can be adapted to various fitness levels helping enhance lower body strength and pelvic stability.

- **Starting Position**: Lie on your back with your feet against the wall and knees bent. Place your arms by your sides, palms facing down.
- **Movement**: Lift your hips into a bridge position and extend one leg toward the ceiling. Be mindful of your breathing.
- **End Position**: Lower the leg back down and switch sides. Perform 2 sets of 8 of repetitions for each leg.

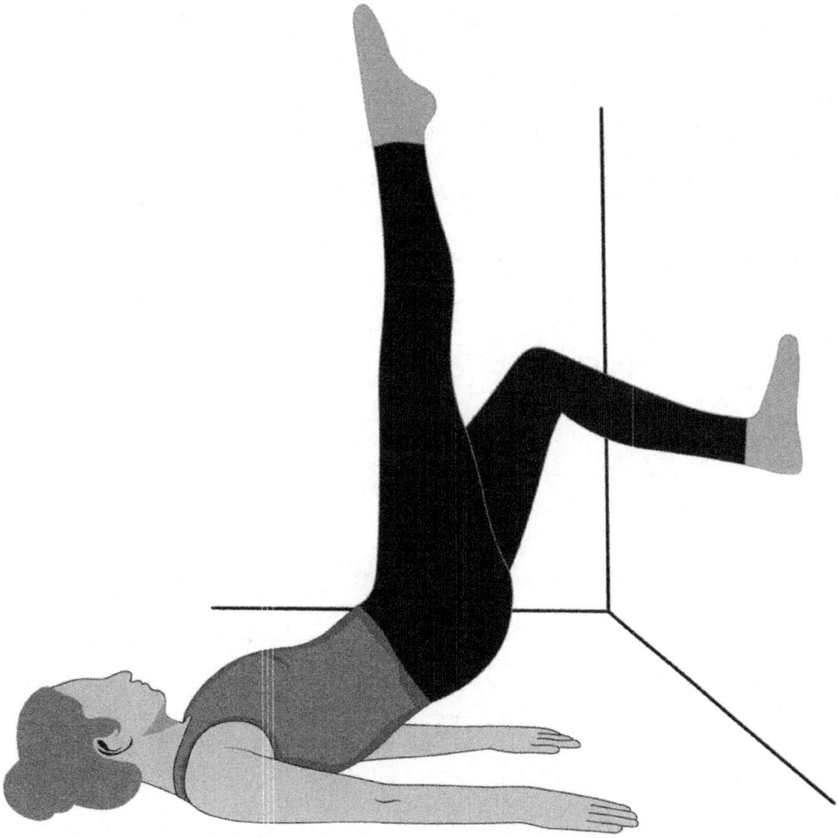

WALL BRIDGE WITH LEG LIFT

Dear esteemed readers,

I am tremendously grateful for the honor of being a part of your fitness journey through this book. Your commitment to staying fit and healthy during your senior years is commendable, and I hope the exercises here have added value.

I would be immensely grateful if you could take a moment to share your thoughts by leaving a review on Amazon.

Your feedback is invaluable, and your review would help me understand your perspective. It would also help other seniors who are starting their own journey.

Thank you for being part of this great community of senior health and fitness.

Toni

Chapter 5:
The 30-Day Calendar

Day 1

Exercise	Notes	Page
Wall Calf Stretch	Hold 5 seconds, repeat 4x	36
Wall Plank	Hold 20 seconds, repeat 3x	40
Wall Leg Raises	10 reps, switch, repeat 2x	44
Wall Roll Down	2 sets of 6 repetitions	48
Hip Flexor Stretch	Hold 15 sec/leg, repeat 2x	52

Day 2

Exercise	Notes	Page
Wall Chest Stretch	Hold 15 sec/side, repeat 3x	37
Wall Side Bend	2 sets of 10 reps each side	41
Wall Marching	3 sets of 60 seconds each	45
Wall Sit	3 sets of 15 seconds each	49
Seated Leg Lifts	2 sets of 10 reps each leg	53

Day 3

Exercise	Notes	Page
Wall Arm Circles	2 sets of 30 seconds each	38
Standing Wall Twist	Repeat full motion 10 times	42
Wall Side Leg Lifts	2 sets of 10 reps each side	46
Leg Press against Wall	2 sets of 8 repetitions	50
Bent Leg Wall Hundred	3 sets of 20 seconds each	54

Remember: Warm up and cool down at the beginning and end of each session. This is crucial for preparing your body to minimize the risk of injury and promote an effective and enjoyable workout.

Day 4

Exercise	Notes	Page
Shoulder Blade Squeeze	2 sets of 10 repetitions	39
Wall Heel Raises	2 sets of 10 repetitions	43
Wall Push Ups	2 sets of 10 repetitions	47
Wall Lunges	2 sets of 8 repetitions	51
Wall Heel Slides	2 sets of 8 reps each leg	55

Day 5

Exercise	Notes	Page
Wall Calf Stretch	Hold 5 seconds, repeat 4x	36
Wall Side Bend	2 sets of 10 reps each side	41
Wall Side Leg Lifts	2 sets of 10 reps each side	46
Wall Roll Down	2 sets of 6 repetitions	48
Wall Hip Bridge	2 sets of 8 repetitions	56

Day 6

Exercise	Notes	Page
Wall Chest Stretch	Hold 15 sec/side, repeat 3x	37
Standing Wall Twist	Repeat full motion 10 times	42
Wall Push Ups	2 sets of 10 repetitions	47
Leg Press against Wall	2 sets of 8 repetitions	50
Wall Bridge w/Leg Lift	2 sets of 8 reps each leg	57

Day 7

Rest Day

Day 8

Exercise	Notes	Page
Wall Calf Stretch	Hold 5 seconds, repeat 4x	36
Wall Plank	Hold 20 seconds, repeat 3x	40
Wall Leg Raises	10 reps, switch, repeat 2x	44
Wall Roll Down	2 sets of 6 repetitions	48
Hip Flexor Stretch	Hold 15 sec/leg, repeat 2x	52

Day 9

Exercise	Notes	Page
Wall Chest Stretch	Hold 15 sec/side, repeat 3x	37
Wall Side Bend	2 sets of 10 reps each side	41
Wall Marching	3 sets of 60 seconds each	45
Wall Sit	3 sets of 15 seconds each	49
Seated Leg Lifts	2 sets of 10 reps each leg	53

Day 10

Exercise	Notes	Page
Wall Arm Circles	2 sets of 30 seconds each	38
Standing Wall Twist	Repeat full motion 10 times	42
Wall Side Leg Lifts	2 sets of 10 reps each side	46
Leg Press against Wall	2 sets of 8 repetitions	50
Bent Leg Wall Hundred	3 sets of 20 seconds each	54

Remember: Warm up and cool down at the beginning and end of each session. This is crucial for preparing your body to minimize the risk of injury and promote an effective and enjoyable workout.

Day 11

Exercise	Notes	Page
Shoulder Blade Squeeze	2 sets of 10 repetitions	39
Wall Heel Raises	2 sets of 10 repetitions	43
Wall Push Ups	2 sets of 10 repetitions	47
Wall Lunges	2 sets of 8 repetitions	51
Wall Heel Slides	2 sets of 8 reps each leg	55

Day 12

Exercise	Notes	Page
Wall Calf Stretch	Hold 5 seconds, repeat 4x	36
Wall Side Bend	2 sets of 10 reps each side	41
Wall Side Leg Lifts	2 sets of 10 reps each side	46
Wall Roll Down	2 sets of 6 repetitions	48
Wall Hip Bridge	2 sets of 8 repetitions	56

Day 13

Exercise	Notes	Page
Wall Chest Stretch	Hold 15 sec/side, repeat 3x	37
Standing Wall Twist	Repeat full motion 10 times	42
Wall Push Ups	2 sets of 10 repetitions	47
Leg Press against Wall	2 sets of 8 repetitions	50
Wall Bridge w/Leg Lift	2 sets of 8 reps each leg	57

Day 14

Rest Day

Day 15

Exercise	Notes	Page
Wall Calf Stretch	**Hold 5 seconds, repeat 4x**	**36**
Wall Plank	**Hold 20 seconds, repeat 3x**	**40**
Wall Leg Raises	**10 reps, switch, repeat 2x**	**44**
Wall Roll Down	**2 sets of 6 repetitions**	**48**
Hip Flexor Stretch	**Hold 15 sec/leg, repeat 2x**	**52**

Day 16

Exercise	Notes	Page
Wall Chest Stretch	**Hold 15 sec/side, repeat 3x**	**37**
Wall Side Bend	**2 sets of 10 reps each side**	**41**
Wall Marching	**3 sets of 60 seconds each**	**45**
Wall Sit	**3 sets of 15 seconds each**	**49**
Seated Leg Lifts	**2 sets of 10 reps each leg**	**53**

Day 17

Exercise	Notes	Page
Wall Arm Circles	**2 sets of 30 seconds each**	**38**
Standing Wall Twist	**Repeat full motion 10 times**	**42**
Wall Side Leg Lifts	**2 sets of 10 reps each side**	**46**
Leg Press against Wall	**2 sets of 8 repetitions**	**50**
Bent Leg Wall Hundred	**3 sets of 20 seconds each**	**54**

Remember: Warm up and cool down at the beginning and end of each session. This is crucial for preparing your body to minimize the risk of injury and promote an effective and enjoyable workout.

Day 18

Exercise	Notes	Page
Shoulder Blade Squeeze	2 sets of 10 repetitions	39
Wall Heel Raises	2 sets of 10 repetitions	43
Wall Push Ups	2 sets of 10 repetitions	47
Wall Lunges	2 sets of 8 repetitions	51
Wall Heel Slides	2 sets of 8 reps each leg	55

Day 19

Exercise	Notes	Page
Wall Calf Stretch	Hold 5 seconds, repeat 4x	36
Wall Side Bend	2 sets of 10 reps each side	41
Wall Side Leg Lifts	2 sets of 10 reps each side	46
Wall Roll Down	2 sets of 6 repetitions	48
Wall Hip Bridge	2 sets of 8 repetitions	56

Day 20

Exercise	Notes	Page
Wall Chest Stretch	Hold 15 sec/side, repeat 3x	37
Standing Wall Twist	Repeat full motion 10 times	42
Wall Push Ups	2 sets of 10 repetitions	47
Leg Press against Wall	2 sets of 8 repetitions	50
Wall Bridge w/Leg Lift	2 sets of 8 reps each leg	57

Day 21

Rest Day

Day 22

Exercise	Notes	Page
Wall Calf Stretch	Hold 5 seconds, repeat 4x	36
Wall Plank	Hold 20 seconds, repeat 3x	40
Wall Leg Raises	10 reps, switch, repeat 2x	44
Wall Roll Down	2 sets of 6 repetitions	48
Hip Flexor Stretch	Hold 15 sec/leg, repeat 2x	52

Day 23

Exercise	Notes	Page
Wall Chest Stretch	Hold 15 sec/side, repeat 3x	37
Wall Side Bend	2 sets of 10 reps each side	41
Wall Marching	3 sets of 60 seconds each	45
Wall Sit	3 sets of 15 seconds each	49
Seated Leg Lifts	2 sets of 10 reps each leg	53

Day 24

Exercise	Notes	Page
Wall Arm Circles	2 sets of 30 seconds each	38
Standing Wall Twist	Repeat full motion 10 times	42
Wall Side Leg Lifts	2 sets of 10 reps each side	46
Leg Press against Wall	2 sets of 8 repetitions	50
Bent Leg Wall Hundred	3 sets of 20 seconds each	54

Remember: Warm up and cool down at the beginning and end of each session. This is crucial for preparing your body to minimize the risk of injury and promote an effective and enjoyable workout.

Day 25

Exercise	Notes	Page
Shoulder Blade Squeeze	2 sets of 10 repetitions	39
Wall Heel Raises	2 sets of 10 repetitions	43
Wall Push Ups	2 sets of 10 repetitions	47
Wall Lunges	2 sets of 8 repetitions	51
Wall Heel Slides	2 sets of 8 reps each leg	55

Day 26

Exercise	Notes	Page
Wall Calf Stretch	Hold 5 seconds, repeat 4x	36
Wall Side Bend	2 sets of 10 reps each side	41
Wall Side Leg Lifts	2 sets of 10 reps each side	46
Wall Roll Down	2 sets of 6 repetitions	48
Wall Hip Bridge	2 sets of 8 repetitions	56

Day 27

Exercise	Notes	Page
Wall Chest Stretch	Hold 15 sec/side, repeat 3x	37
Standing Wall Twist	Repeat full motion 10 times	42
Wall Push Ups	2 sets of 10 repetitions	47
Leg Press against Wall	2 sets of 8 repetitions	50
Wall Bridge w/Leg Lift	2 sets of 8 reps each leg	57

Day 28

Rest Day

Day 29

Exercise	Notes	Page
Wall Calf Stretch	**Hold 5 seconds, repeat 4x**	**36**
Wall Plank	**Hold 20 seconds, repeat 3x**	**40**
Wall Leg Raises	**10 reps, switch, repeat 2x**	**44**
Wall Roll Down	**2 sets of 6 repetitions**	**48**
Hip Flexor Stretch	**Hold 15 sec/leg, repeat 2x**	**52**

Day 30

Exercise	Notes	Page
Wall Chest Stretch	**Hold 15 sec/side, repeat 3x**	**38**
Wall Side Bend	**2 sets of 10 reps each side**	**42**
Wall Marching	**3 sets of 60 seconds each**	**46**
Wall Sit	**3 sets of 15 seconds each**	**50**
Seated Leg Lifts	**2 sets of 10 reps each leg**	**54**

Congratulations on completing this 30-Day Wall Pilates program! Your hard work has paid off, and the satisfaction of reaching this milestone is truly commendable. As you look back and reflect on the last 30 days, consider the beneficial impact on your physical and mental well-being. Let this sense of accomplishment fuel your motivation to continue with the momentum for the next 30 days. Continue challenging yourself and stay focused.

Keep going – you've got this!

Chapter 6:

Good Nutrition

Wall Pilates and Good Nutrition

The importance of good nutrition cannot be overstated as you embark on your Wall Pilates journey. Just as the body relies on precise movements against the wall for strength and flexibility, it also requires a well-balanced diet for sustained energy, muscle recovery, and overall vitality. A mindful and tailored approach to nutrition becomes essential to support the unique needs of seniors and optimize the benefits of Wall Pilates.

Here are 9 ways how a holistic approach that integrates Wall Pilates with an excellent nutritional plan contributes to overall well-being:

1. Enhanced Mobility and Joint Health

Wall Pilates emphasizes controlled movements and joint mobilization to support enhanced mobility for seniors. Pairing this with a nutrition plan rich in anti-inflammatory foods contributes to joint health. For example, foods like fatty fish, walnuts, and flaxseeds contain omega-3 fatty acids with anti-inflammatory properties, potentially reducing joint discomfort and supporting overall mobility.

2. Mind-Body Connection

Both Wall Pilates and mindful nutrition practices cultivate a solid mind-body connection. The deliberate movements against the wall and the focus on breath awareness in Pilates promote mindfulness. Similarly, remember mindful eating practices, such as making good food choices when going to the grocery store or going out to eat at a restaurant. Also, be aware of hunger and fullness cues, which enhances the connection between seniors and their nutrition. This approach fosters a positive relationship with both movement and nutrition.

3. Stress Reduction and Mental Clarity

Engaging in Wall Pilates and adopting a nutrition plan that includes mood-boosting nutrients contribute to stress reduction and mental clarity for seniors. Physical activity, such as Pilates, releases endorphins, promoting well-being. Nutrient-dense foods, notably those rich in omega-3 fatty acids, antioxidants, and B vitamins, support brain health and cognitive function, reducing stress and allowing for mental clarity.

4. Weight Management and Body Composition

The combination of Wall Pilates and nutrition is effective for seniors in managing weight and optimizing body composition. Pilates aids muscle tone, flexibility, and cardiovascular fitness, while a balanced and nutrient-dense diet supports healthy weight maintenance. This encourages a positive body image and sustainable lifestyle habits.

5. Sustainable Energy Levels

Seniors benefit from sustained energy levels, especially during and after Wall Pilates sessions. A nutrition plan that includes a mix of complex carbohydrates, lean proteins, and healthy fats ensures a steady release of energy. Coupled with the cardiovascular and muscular benefits of Pilates, it contributes to sustained vitality throughout daily activities.

6. Promotion of Bone Health

Wall Pilates exercises, which often involve weight-bearing movements, contribute to bone health for seniors. As we age, we lose nutrients and minerals from our bones, such as calcium. Good nutrition and exercise help seniors preserve their bone density and prevent fractures.

7. Hydration for Overall Vitality

Hydration is a foundational aspect of both Pilates and nutrition for seniors. Proper fluid intake supports joint lubrication, temperature regulation, and overall bodily functions. Aging individuals may have an increased risk of dehydration due to changes in thirst perception and kidney function. Seniors should prioritize hydration before, during, and after Wall Pilates sessions and throughout the day as part of their comprehensive approach to well-being.

8. Digestive Health

Incorporating fiber-rich foods and probiotics into the nutrition plan supports digestive health for seniors. Whole grains, fruits, vegetables, and fermented foods contribute to a thriving gut microbiome. This is complemented by the controlled movements in Wall Pilates, which can aid digestion and nutrient absorption.

9. Positive Lifestyle Habits and Longevity

The integration of Wall Pilates and nutrition encourages positive habits and contributes to longevity. Regular physical activity and a healthful diet are foundational pillars for long-term well-being. This integrated approach fosters practices supporting health and vitality throughout aging.

Nutritional Foundations for Seniors

Some essential nutritional foundations for seniors engaging in Wall Pilates include:

1. Nutrient-Dense Diet

Seniors benefit from a nutrient-dense diet rich in vitamins, minerals, and antioxidants. Fruits, vegetables, lean proteins, whole grains, and healthy fats form the foundation of a balanced and nourishing diet. These foods provide essential nutrients that support bone health, muscle function, and overall immune function. Seniors should focus on consuming various colorful fruits and vegetables to ensure a broad spectrum of nutrients avoiding processed and packaged foods.

2. Balanced Macronutrients

Achieving a balance of macronutrients, carbohydrates, proteins, and fats is crucial for seniors. Carbohydrates provide the necessary energy for physical activity, proteins support muscle maintenance and repair, and healthy fats contribute to overall cellular function. A balanced mix of these macronutrients supports sustained energy levels and recovery.

3. Adequate Protein Intake

Protein becomes increasingly crucial for seniors to maintain muscle mass and help with recovery. It's vital to include protein-rich foods like lean meats, poultry, fish, dairy, eggs, and plant-based sources like legumes and tofu. Protein intake should be distributed throughout the day, including in meals and snacks, to support muscle protein synthesis.

Pre-Workout Nutrition

Seniors should consider a well-balanced meal or snack before engaging in Wall Pilates to ensure optimal performance and energy levels. Pre-workout snacks can include a banana with nut butter or yogurt with granola.

Post-Workout Nutrition

The post-workout period is critical for seniors to replenish glycogen stores and support muscle recovery. Consuming a balanced combination of carbohydrates and protein within the first hour after Wall Pilates is beneficial. Options include a protein smoothie with fruits or a balanced meal with lean protein and whole grains.

Supplementation Considerations

Seniors may need good quality supplementation based on individual requirements and potential nutrient deficiencies. Common considerations include vitamin D for bone health, calcium for bone density, and omega-3 fatty acids for joint and cardiovascular and brain health. Ensure you consult a healthcare professional or registered dietitian for guidance on appropriate supplementation based on your needs and activity level.

Bone Health Support

Seniors are often concerned about bone health, and proper nutrition is vital in supporting and preserving bone density. Adequate calcium and vitamin D intake is essential. Foods like leafy greens, dairy products, fatty fish, and fortified cereals contribute to these nutrients. Seniors should also focus on foods that are rich in vitamin K, magnesium, and phosphorus for comprehensive bone health support.

Antioxidant-Rich Foods

Incorporating foods rich in antioxidants in your diet can help combat oxidative stress and inflammation associated with aging. Berries, dark leafy greens, nuts, seeds, and colorful vegetables are excellent sources of antioxidants. These foods contribute to overall cellular health and may help mitigate the impact of aging on the body.

Gut Health Considerations

Maintaining a healthy gut is essential for seniors' overall well-being. Ensure you eat fiber-rich foods like fruits, whole grains, vegetables, and probiotic-rich foods like yogurt and kefir to maintain digestive health. Seniors should also prioritize a diverse range of fiber sources to promote a thriving gut microbiome.

Implementing a Holistic Approach to Good Nutrition

Here's how you can implement a holistic approach that combines mindful nutrition with the transformative practice of Wall Pilates to enhance your overall well-being:

1. Consultation with Healthcare Professionals

Always consult healthcare professionals to assess your health status before starting any fitness or nutrition plan. Obtain clearance from your healthcare provider to ensure that both Wall Pilates and changes in your nutrition plan are safe and appropriate for your unique needs and any underlying health conditions.

2. Customized Nutrition Plan

Work with a registered dietitian to create a customized nutrition plan tailored to your specific requirements as a senior. It should consider age, gender, activity level, medical history, and dietary preferences.

3. Practice Mindful Eating

Ultimate mindful eating practices to enhance your relationship with food. Mindful eating promotes better digestion, improved nutrient absorption, while giving you a greater appreciation for the nourishing qualities of food.

4. Regular Assessments and Adjustments

Periodically reassess your nutrition and this Wall Pilates plan in collaboration with healthcare professionals. You may need to adjust the plans depending on your health, fitness level, or goal changes.

Celebration of Progress

Celebrate milestones and progress in both your nutrition and Wall Pilates journey. Recognize the positive changes in energy levels, flexibility, and overall well-being. Fitness is a lifelong journey, and acknowledging achievements will help reinforce a positive and sustainable lifestyle.

A Final Word

Seeing Results

You've got the know-how, you've got the tools, and you have a 30-day workout plan. All that's left is for you to commit to the process and stick to it for 30 days to start seeing results. It goes without saying that Wall Pilates is an effective and accessible exercise method for seniors like you looking to maintain and improve an active and healthy lifestyle. This type of Pilates leverages the support of a wall, providing stability and balance for older adults while promoting strength, flexibility, and overall well-being.

Wall Pilates is tailored to meet the unique needs of seniors. The wall support reduces the risk of falls, making it an ideal exercise method. It also presents a myriad of benefits for seniors. Wall Pilates places a significant focus on core engagement, aiding in the development and maintenance of core strength. This is particularly beneficial for older adults as a strong core contributes to better balance and stability. The controlled and deliberate movements in Wall Pilates also promotes flexibility, helping you maintain a full range of motion in your joints. This is crucial for activities of daily living and can alleviate stiffness associated with aging.

As a low-impact exercise, Wall Pilates is gentle on joints, making it suitable for seniors with arthritis or other mobility issues. It offers an effective way to stay active without putting undue stress on the body. It's crucial to ensure you learn about breathing correctly during movements, as rhythmic, deliberate breathing techniques facilitate physical exertion and contribute to a deeper mind-body connection. Breathing in Wall Pilates is not merely a physiological necessity but a tool for enhancing the effectiveness of each exercise.

Another principle of Wall Pilates is control, and it involves performing each exercise in a deliberate, controlled, and conscious way. Controlled movements lie at the heart of Wall Pilates, emphasizing the intentional execution of each exercise. The wall becomes a partner in this pursuit, offering stability and resistance that demand precise control. Whether engaging in standing exercises or incorporating the wall for support in mat-based movements, practitioners focus on the art of controlled motion.

You can also promote stability, balance, and control through centering. Centering is about mental focus. You're encouraged to maintain a deep sense of concentration where you perform each movement with precision and control. The mental aspect of centering reinforces the mind-body connection, turning Wall Pilates into a mindful practice that fosters an integral approach to health and fitness.

Establish good form to set the foundation for the entire workout and reduce the risk of strain or injury. Gradually progress through your routine instead of making sudden, jerky movements. Listen to your body and adjust the workout intensity based on how you feel. Don't shy away from modifying movements or stopping if necessary. Also, ensure you have proper footwear and attire that doesn't restrict movement. Ensure sufficient clearance around the wall where you'll perform Wall Pilates exercises. Remove any obstacles or furniture that may impede your movements. Optimal lighting is essential for safety and focus during the warm-up, so keep the space well-lit, either with natural or artificial light. Proper lighting reduces the risk of tripping or missteps.

An effective warm-up for Wall Pilates should encompass various preparation techniques that gradually engage the muscles and increase the heart rate. The goal is to prepare the body and mind for the specific demands of Wall Pilates exercises and lay the groundwork for a more profound and effective workout.

It's also vital to ensure you maintain good nutritional practices when undertaking Wall Pilates. A well-balanced diet is necessary for sustained energy, muscle recovery, and overall vitality. Hydration is a foundational aspect of both Pilates and nutrition for seniors. Proper fluid intake supports joint lubrication, temperature regulation, and general bodily functions. Seniors should prioritize hydration before, during, and after Wall Pilates sessions and throughout the day as part of their comprehensive approach to well-being. A nutrient-dense diet rich in vitamins, minerals, and antioxidants provides essential nutrients that support bone health, muscle function, and overall immune function. Consider a well-balanced meal or snack before and after engaging in Wall Pilates to ensure optimal performance and energy levels, replenish glycogen stores, and support muscle recovery.

Wall Pilates together with a good nutrition plan is an effective combination to help you achieve your fitness and health goals. Consulting a healthcare professional or working with a registered diet specialist to create a customized nutrition plan tailored to your specific requirements would be a great compliment to your Wall Pilates practice. You can also practice mindful eating practices that promote better digestion, improved nutrient absorption, and a greater appreciation for food. Stress management practices like meditation are also essential for complementing the physical benefits of Wall Pilates and nutrition. Emotional well-being contributes to a positive mindset and resilience as you get older.

"Remember to Celebrate Milestones and Progress in Your Wall Pilates Journey."

Recognize the positive changes in energy levels, flexibility, and overall well-being. The key to getting the most out of Wall Pilates is consistency. It is recommended to practice Wall Pilates exercises regularly, at least three to four times per week, to see noticeable changes in strength, flexibility, and balance. We highly recommend using the calendar provided in chapter 5 in this book. Additionally, it is essential to use proper form and engage the core muscles throughout the exercises for maximum benefit and to reduce injury risk.

Another critical aspect of continuing Wall Pilates is to challenge yourself. As you get stronger and more attuned to the exercises, you can adjust the intensity and duration of your workouts gradually. For example, you can try adding weights or resistance bands to your movements or increasing the number of repetitions for each exercise.

With all of this said, here's a heartfelt thank you for adding this book to your quest for a healthier and better you. I trust this book will take your fitness to the next level and will open your mind about the possibilities of a healthy, active, and exciting life as a senior.

In health and fitness,
Toni Avalos

Dear esteemed readers,

Once again, I am tremendously grateful for the honor of being a part of your fitness journey through this book. Your commitment to staying fit and healthy during your senior years is commendable, and I hope the exercises here have added value.

I would be immensely grateful if you could take a moment to share your thoughts by leaving a review on Amazon.

Your feedback is invaluable, and your review would help me understand your perspective. It would also help other seniors who are starting their own journey.

Thank you for being part of this great community of senior health and fitness!

Find Resources and Support at:

StrongandAgeless.com

SCAN ME

All Titles in the Strong & Ageless Series:

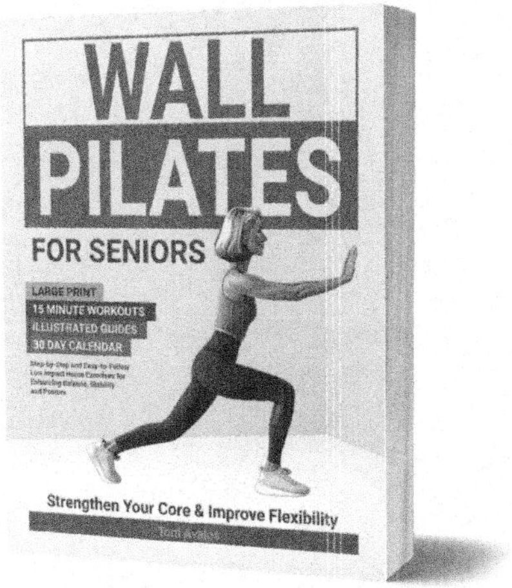

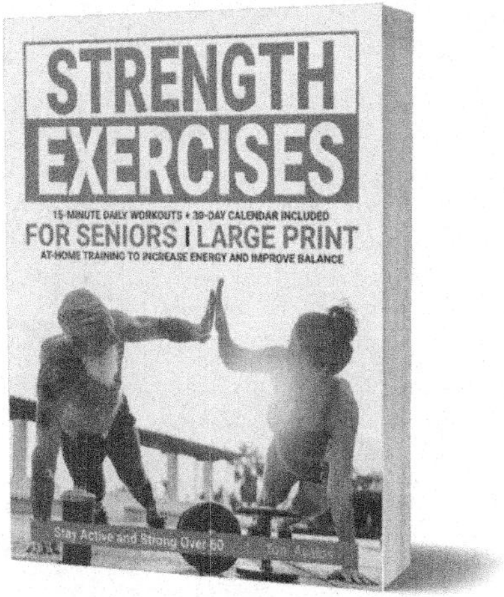

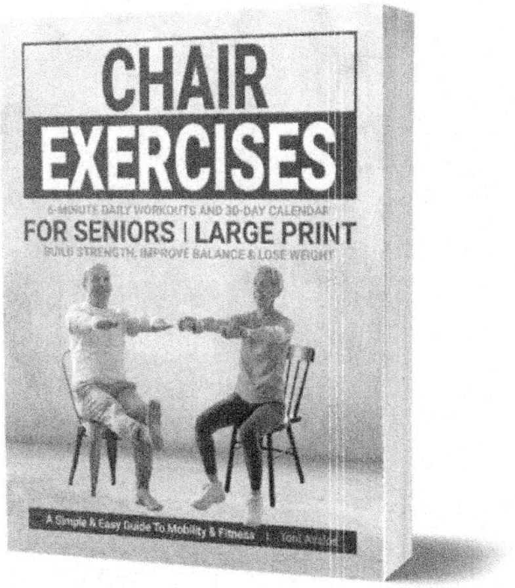

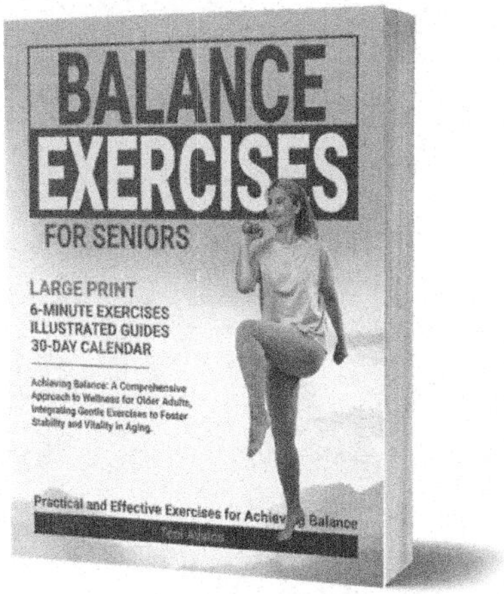

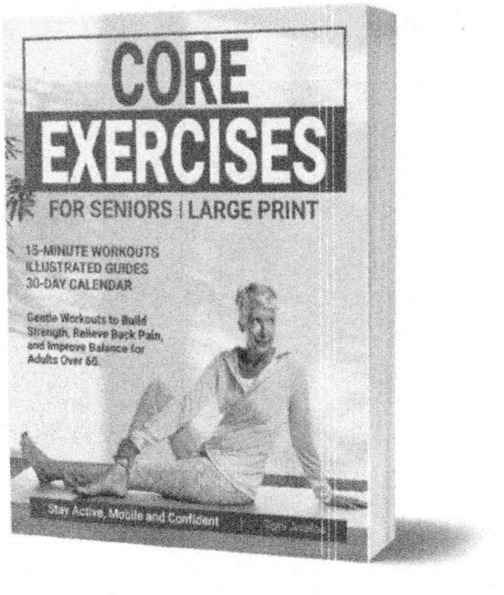

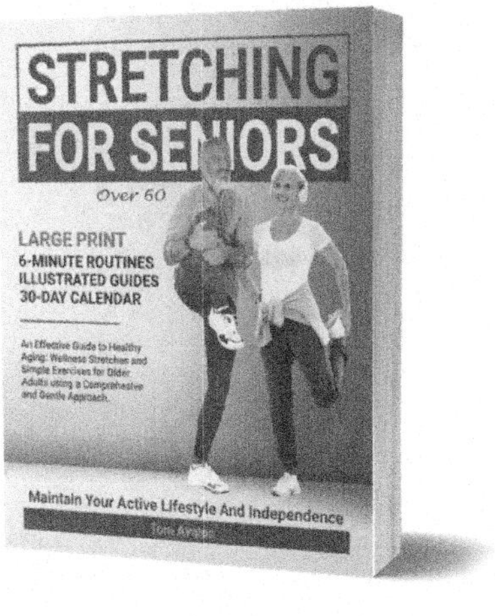

StrongandAgeless.com

Printed in Dunstable, United Kingdom

80015510R00051